# Changing Mental
# Health Services

D1302113

# Changing Mental Health Services
## The politics and policy

*Tom Butler*

**CHAPMAN & HALL**

London · Glasgow · New York · Tokyo · Melbourne · Madras

**Published by Chapman & Hall, 2–6 Boundary Row, London SE1 8HN**

Chapman & Hall, 2–6 Boundary Row, London SE1 8HN, UK

Blackie Academic & Professional, Wester Cleddens Road, Bishopbriggs, Glasgow G64 2NZ, UK

Chapman & Hall, 29 West 35th Street, New York NY10001, USA

Chapman & Hall Japan, Thomson Publishing Japan, Hirakawacho Nemoto Building, 6F, 1–7–11 Hirakawa-cho, Chiyoda-ku, Tokyo 102, Japan

Chapman & Hall Australia, Thomas Nelson Australia, 102 Dodds Street, South Melbourne, Victoria 3205, Australia

Chapman & Hall India, R. Seshadri, 32 Second Main Road, CIT East, Madras 600 035, India

First edition 1993

© 1993  Tom Butler

Typeset in 10/12 Palatino by Mews Photosetting, Beckenham, Kent
Printed in Great Britain by St Edmundsbury Press, Bury St Edmunds, Suffolk

ISBN 0 412 40500 8      1 56593 035 5 (USA)

# Contents

# Acknowledgements

The ideas explored here owe much to colleagues and friends and I would like to thank the following people in the Department of Psychiatry at the Manchester Royal Infirmary and the University Department; Professor Francis Creed, Dr Keith Bridges, Professor Peter Huxley, Dr Madeleine Osborn, and John Riley, Rehabilitation Services Manager. I would also like to thank Dr Phil Thomas of the Meirionydd Community Mental Health Team; Professor Howard Goldman and Susan Ridgely of Mental Health Policy Studies, University of Maryland who helped to improve my understanding of issues in American community mental health care; Dr Richard Warner, Medical Director, Boulder Mental Health Centre and Ernest Sessa, Executive Director of the Pennsylvania Health Care Cost Containment Council for help with sources and material.

The person I am most indebted to is my wife Marion Butler whose patience, good sense and encouragement helped me enormously in writing this book.

Any errors in this book are, as always, my own responsibility.

# Preface

The idea for this book arose out of the experience of managing mental health services in inner-city Manchester. The book is an attempt to make sense of the changes in mental health policy and practice *within the context* of the wider reforms in health and social care in Britain.

This book is about the ways society has responded to people with mental illness through changing social policy over time. It is about the way in which attitudes, public policy and professional practice has changed in mental health policy and provision. It is aimed at those people who are undergoing professional training or education in the mental health field and who want to look at issues of policy and practice in a social, political and historical context.

Mention 'mental illness' or 'the mentally ill' in ordinary conversation and it conjures up powerful and conflicting images. These include pictures of people incarcerated in isolated institutions; pathetic sad individuals, incoherent and impoverished people talking loudly in public places, lonely people cut off from society or those whose behaviour is dangerous or volatile. These stereotypes serve to reinforce the view that there is a single group of people called 'the mentally ill' who deserve pity or fear in equal measure. These convenient stereotypes make complex relationships and personal histories easier to classify, categorize and dismiss. The alternative is less tidy and more uncomfortable as it involves having to understand the individual's own history, family life, ambitions, feelings, and attitudes separate from his or her illness. Much of the experience of people with mental illness has been as a troubled and occasionally troublesome minority at the margins of mainstream society.

The language we use to describe either 'mental illness' or 'mental health' services is itself loaded with meaning and belief. Much of the language of the past such as 'lunacy' and 'madness' is now denounced as stigmatizing and we now refer to 'patients, 'clients' or 'service-users', just as 'mental illness services' is giving way to the more positive but inexact 'mental health services'. The changes in the language in part reflects a change in social attitude towards people with mental illness as well as the emergence of interest groups which seek to represent the views of service-users. It is only by looking at the way in which attitudes, policies and practice has changed over time that we can begin to understand the way in which society has *developed* public policy and professional practice. This emergence of public policy has involved changes in attitude, policy and practice which have been uneven, contradictory and repetitive; crosscut with scandal, innovation and frustration. Perhaps the one recurring theme in the development of public policy and services for people with mental illness is the way in which long-standing problems, remedies and solutions have been identified, rejected and re-discovered from time to time. There is little that is genuinely novel and innovative in policy and practice except for the label we attach to it.

The approach taken in this book will look at a range of differing strategies which have been employed to provide for the people with mental illness. These strategies have been seen as 'solutions' to the social problem of mental illness and have ranged from the use of containment in institutions through to the much publicized 'care in the community' policies. This book explores the origins of these policies and examines the consequences for the professionals and service-users alike. Particular attention is given to the contrasts between the rhetoric which introduced new policies and practices and the experience of patients and staff who lived with the consequences.

Social policy is one way of expressing political beliefs and social and public policy for mental health is no exception. In the nineteenth century mental health policy was an important political topic as it was one example of the newly developing role of central and local government which regulated the lives of individual citizens. For most of the twentieth century public policy on mental health has been represented as if it developed in a political vacuum. This book seeks to challenge this view and argues that social policy is necessarily political, especially when it deals with issues such as public expenditure and the loss of liberty. The changes in the National Health Service which were introduced at the beginning of the 1990s highlighted the intensely political character of social policy and health provision. One part of this process was to establish a new pattern of service organization and provision for mental health both in hospital and community services. Many of the proposed changes have been introduced because they are perceived to be desirable, rather than being rooted in the experience of the professionals or service-users who seek coherent, consistent, appropriate and accessible services to meet a range of short-term and long-term needs.

This book also examines the reforms of the National Health Service and the role of Social Services Departments in order to understand how these changes came about and the implications for mental health services in Britain. In order to see the practical effects of the changes in national social policy there is a short case study of the experience of managing change and the provision of mental health services in inner city Manchester in the early 1990s. By way of contrast the book also includes an account of some of the new mental health services which have been developed in America and which suggest alternative and innovative ways of organizing and providing services.

For over 30 years there has been a rather unproductive debate within mental health services in Britain about understanding needs and providing appropriate services. Much of this debate has been either to defend hospital care or to promote community provision. The result all too often has been to polarize services and limit the development of a comprehensive range of services to meet the needs of the population.

This book attempts to look at the issue in a new way which pulls together a number of disparate strands. In particular it proposes an alternative approach to the planning and management of services. This is based on a decision-making process which seeks to involve the key stake-holders, including the service-user, in order to identify individual need. The approach also attempts to establish the capacity of the services to meet these needs and records the shortfall.

The starting point for this process is an attempt to engage purchasers of service, users and professionals in establishing a set of shared values for the provision of mental health services locally. The approach allows individual care planning information to be aggregated in such a way that it may serve to improve the understanding of the needs of the local population for mental health services overall. Equally this alternative approach attempts to establish the staff development needs of multi-agency teams in light of the experience of planning services for individual users. The development of services is seen all too often only in terms of an increase in buildings and plant, whereas the most important resource is the staff themselves. If individual care planning for mental health service-users is to be developed then the service-providers also need to be developed in parallel. The process described in Chapter 9 is a search for an alternative way of working which allows agencies to find a common framework within which to work. It begins to set out a way of identifying the resource needs of local services including staff development, as a consequences of providing services, not as an afterthought.

The approach described above is a framework in which to plan and deliver services, it is *not* a prescription which can be mechanically applied. It does not assume any particular model of service or organizational structure as it is a process for developing services. It is a challenge to the traditional way of working which has resulted in fragmented services for service-users and professionals alike. One of the likely consequences of this approach is that it would be possible to have access to two key sets of data which up to now have been notable by their absence. First, an accurate record of the services delivered and shortfall in provision and, second, a commitment by professionals to focus their work on producing clear outcomes which improve the quality of life for service-users.

Establishing a system of mental health provision which records the impact of services on the quality of life of service-users is one way of cutting through the political rhetoric and unfulfilled promises made by successive governments. To those who work in and depend upon mental health services the last three decades have been a story of fragmented services, unfulfilled promises and empty rhetoric.

Tom Butler
Department of Psychiatry
Manchester Royal Infirmary

# 1

## The Victorian legacy of the mentally ill

### INSTITUTIONS AND ATTITUDES: THE PROBLEM OF DOING GOOD

This chapter opens with a look at the past. It examines some of the ideas and practices which shaped services today. It will be argued that unless we have an understanding of where our policies, practices, and resources came from, it is impossible to tackle the problems of today in an informed way. Good practice does not come from carers following procedures in a mechanical and an unthinking way. Rather, it is essential to understand the issues which have shaped the world we work in. Procedures are important if they are linked to setting and evaluating clear standards. By themselves procedures do not ensure that good-quality, appropriate services are provided. It will be argued in this book that setting clear standards is important if we are concerned with demonstrating competence, but that using procedures slavishly, i.e. mere rule-following, can stifle innovation.

For those people who work in mental health services today it is easy to look at services in the past as being at best, patronizing and, at worst, cruel. It is often uncomfortable to look at the impact and influence of earlier services on our policies, practice and attitudes. Many clients and patients were treated in ways that we now regard as archaic or simply wrong.

It is important that we do not confuse the policies, provision and approaches of the past with the problems of today. It will be shown in this chapter that the population of the large nineteenth century asylums were different from those people who use mental health services today. Many of the institutions still continue to be used largely for long-stay, elderly patients admitted in another era. The experience for the majority of people using mental health services in 1990s Britain does not involve hospital admission let alone a long stay in institutional care. But the old asylums still cast a powerful shadow over public attitudes and instil caution and fear. The paradox of the situation is that, despite the powerful emotions produced by the old hospitals, there have been repeated examples throughout the 1980s and early 1990s of local public resistance to the resettlement of long-stay patients which followed from the government programme of hospital contraction and closure.

The way society provides for people with mental illness in Britain has changed significantly over the last 250 years. However these changes have not appeared as the gradual unfolding of a shared vision of policy and provision for people with mental illness. Rather there have been a variety of strategies which have held sway for a period and have in turn been challenged by alternative approaches. It will be argued in this book that since the middle of the eighteenth century there have been eight dominant stratgies which have claimed to provide 'solutions' to the social problem of mental illness. These eight strategies reflect the influence of differing interest groups on those politicians and advisers who drafted public policy. The eight dominant ideas which have shaped policy and practice are set out chronologically below:

| | |
|---|---|
| 1744–1845 | Informal provision made by the local parish using the workhouse and the private madhouses. |
| 1845–1890 | Building of the new public asylums. |
| 1890–1930 | New lunacy laws introduced which required the use of certification before admission to the asylums. |
| 1930–1948 | The psychiatrist and a medical model of mental ilness increasingly accepted. |
| 1948–1954 | New welfare policies developed for health and social care. |
| 1954–1975 | Introduction and use of the new technology of drugs. |

1975–1990    Care in the community forms the basis for public policy.

1991 to date    The market place introduced as a shaper of health and social care with an increased emphasis on inter-agency cooperation and clarification of function.

Clearly this chronological list is a summary of complex and powerful shifts and changes both in society and in the policies established by successive generations. The dates shown are not exact in the sense that each approach started and stopped at precisely the date shown. The point being made here is that it is possible to unravel the major strands in the emergence of public policy directed at people with mental illness and identify the approaches which dominated the thinking of officials and professionals in particular periods. Such an approach can help our understanding of the origins of current policy and practice by setting it in the context of the contemporary political, professional and economic ideas. The way in which people with mental illness are provided for reflects the dominant values of society as a whole. It is only by looking at changes in policy and practice in a social context can the broader picture be appreciated. Without such an approach our ability to understand changes in policies and practices which effect people with mental illness becomes either a justification for current thinking or an unintelligible collision of beliefs and approaches.

## ASYLUMS, STEREOTYPING AND DETENTION

It will be argued in this chapter that we are living with a powerful legacy from the nineteenth century which shapes much of our ideas and practice. Such is the impact of the nineteenth century legacy that much of the work of current mental health services is based on either (i) the pull produced by practices which grew up in the Victorian asylum or (ii) the push which resulted from the reaction against institutional care. The legacy of the Victorian asylum and the nineteenth century policies on lunacy have proven to be remarkably resilient. It will be argued here that the legacy of the past has three major strands:

1. the continued use of the large Victorian hospitals which largely house reducing numbers of long-term elderly patients;

2.  the enduring and popular stereotyping of people with
    mental illness as pitiful or dangerous;
3.  the right of professionals to detain compulsorily people
    with mental illness if required.

The creation of the asylums in the nineteenth century was
the result of a reform campaign which not only produced new
types of buildings to house people deemed to be 'mad'; it also
created an institutional base for the development of new
professions who claimed expert knowledge in the care and
control of people with mental illness. The legacy of the
nineteenth century continues as a powerful influence on
contemporary policy and practice as it produced the buildings
which are associated with mental illness and the professions
who cared for those people who were resident.

One of the major themes of this book is the way in which
the same set of problems, issues and solutions tend to recur
time and time again. On each occasion new approaches are
developed which seek to find novel policies and practices to
respond to persistent problems. The eight 'solutions' to the
problem of mental illness bear witness to this process as each
in turn took as their starting point the deficiencies of the earlier
approach.

It is comforting to take the popular view that in the past
the way in which the mentally ill were treated was simply cruel
and uncaring. It is even more comfortable for us to contrast
past policies and practices with current services. The picture
we like to present of our approaches and services today is to
characterize them as comprehensive, scientific and humane.
The reality for those who work in and live with services today
does not fit this picture. For much of the time patients, their
families and professionals operate in a world which lies in the
shadow of the asylums. The reality for many people is that
the large old hospitals set on the fringes of the cities and towns
have persisted. The development of new services takes place
in the context of the continued existence of the asylums.
Perhaps even more concerning is the degree to which the ideas
that being mentally ill and being detained in hospital are
synonymous has persisted.

The recognition that the role and work of the asylums was
more to do with the containment of patients than the delivery

of therapies was a significant, but limited step in changing the way society provided for the mentally ill. Much of the last 40 years has been spent in trying to reduce the scale of the large old hospitals and to provide services to the mentally ill in a more accessible and less restrictive way. One of the themes which will be explored later is the changing experience and expectations of people who use our services today.

In the past it was patients and staff who were locked up in the large old hospitals on the fringes of towns and cities. Now it is the resources which are tied up in a system which has produced public scandal and private stigma. It is argued in this book that past policies, practices and attitudes continue to have a profound influence on the way that society regards mental illness and the mentally ill. At the most practical level we can see many of the old buildings which continue to be used for the delivery of patient services. But the level of influence is much more subtle and pervasive than just the use of outmoded buildings. The roles and relationships between differing occupational groups such as doctors, nurses and local government officials were founded in the nineteenth century and have developed and persisted. Equally the emergence of social policies on mental health appeared initially as vagrancy and lunacy laws in the eighteenth and nineteenth centuries. Current legislation which deals with the mentally ill shares the same pedigree as the lunacy laws in that it links mental illness with compulsory detention in hospital. The major difference in current practice is that compulsion is used for a small minority of patients whereas by the end of the last century it was the way into services for the mentally ill. If we are to have a better understanding of the ways in which current services developed then we need to take some time to understand both the roots of those services and the legacy which persists. This means looking in a little more detail at past problems faced by those who managed and provided services for people with mental illness.

In the early nineteenth century, before the development of the asylums in each of the English counties, 'care' of the mentally ill was informally organized. With the emergence of the asylum there appeared a single solution to a range of complex medical, social and economic problems. The ayslums were successful in fulfilling the task given to them by society. Their role was to detain those people whom society judged to be incapable of caring for themselves because they were a social nuisance, an economic burden or a danger to others.

The Victorian response to the mentally ill was to deal with them in the same way as other groups such as orphans, the aged, offenders and the disabled. A range of separate institutions was created to provide for those who were categorized as being mad, bad or incapable. The institutions operated within a legal framework and a number of specialist occupations associated with the workings of the asylum emerged. In particular this was evident in the use of certification and subsequent detention of patients. In two key respects the asylums differed from other forms of institutional provision. First, the asylums were lead by doctors who became involved in the management of the mentally ill. Second, the asylums pre-dated many of the other types of institution, therefore acting as a model of provision which could be applied to other groups of people who became dependent on the local parish or county.

The asylums grew rapidly in the nineteenth century and with the support of legislation, so did the number of people classified as 'lunatics'. This raises a number of interesting questions about the role of the institutions and the way in which those people incapable of caring for themselves were dealt with. After 1845 each county was required to build and run its own asylum, as a result the number of institutions available to the magistrate was transformed. By 1854 there were 37 public asylums and 181 private madhouses being supervised by the Commissioners in Lunacy as the central government inspectorate was called. By 1900 there were 77 asylums, each with an average population of 961 patients.

But who were these reformers who achieved so much in terms of persuading government to build the asylums and to introduce the lunacy laws? Many of those who became involved in the reform movement were involved in other issues of social reform or were active in religious organizations independent of the established church. The late eighteenth and early nineteenth centuries proved to be a period of intense activity for those involved in the reform movement. Some changes had been made to the vagrancy laws which covered most of the mentally disturbed. Following an investigation by a parliamentary select committee in 1807 a new piece of legislation was passed which made the provision for lunatics the specific responsibility of local Justices of the Peace. The select committee membership included notable reformers such as Wynn, Wilberforce and Whitbread. Many other well-meaning people were drawn into the issue of the care of lunatics. In York Godfrey Higgins a local magistrate investigated the death of a young Quaker girl in the York asylum. In 1792 William Tuke one of the most famous of the reformers became involved in the plight of detained lunatics. He investigated the conditions of St Luke's Hospital as part of his work with the Society of Friends. From this work there arose an alternative view on how to provide for the daily care of the mentally ill through 'moral treatment'.

The list of investigations, parliamentary enquiries and scandals associated with the asylums and old hospitals is extensive in the period from the end of the eighteenth and up to the middle of the nineteenth century. Some hospitals became subject to continuous rumours and enquiries and the most notorious of these was Bethlem Hospital in London. Parliamentary select committees between 1814 and 1816 looked at York, Nottingham and Bethlem. Out of these visits there arose a catalogue of cases which detailed examples of cruel treatment, although the patients names such as Hannah Mills of St Lukes's and William Norris of Bethlem are now all but forgotten. What also emerged from these enquiries was a clear leader for the reform movement to change the provision for the mentally ill. Anthony Ashley Cooper, 7th Earl of Shaftesbury effectively became the champion of the lunacy reform movement for almost two-thirds of the nineteenth century. Shaftesbury saw in the major reforms of 1845 which required each county to build and provide specific provision for the mentally ill. His work covered the most significant period of the century from the 1830s to 1885 which saw the shift from the creation of the asylums to prevent cruel treatment, to the introduction of the lunacy laws which ensured that lunatics had to be legally certified before being admitted.

It is important to understand why the nineteenth century proved to be ripe for the social reforms proposed by those who sought to change policy and practice associated with lunacy. There is no single explanation which can completely satisfy this question. Those people prominent in the reform of the lunacy laws had a vision of public institutions as practical examples of good government which could be as well regulated as the new industries. The vehicle to achieve this managed and regulated system was the new public asylum. The staff who led these institutions especially the doctors, built their speciality within the institutions and claimed expert knowledge in the field of madness. Private misery was managed in public institutions which were built on a grand scale and which proved to be signficant employers in the local economy. The implications of the reform movement and the unintended consequences of the reformers' actions will be explored later in this chapter. Before looking at the impact of the movement to reform the policy, practice and provision for people classed as 'lunatics' it is necessary to look more closely at who these people were.

In his study of Victorian provision for the mentally ill, Scull (1979) looked at the numbers of people detained in the asylums. This analsyis showed that in 1844 there were less than 21 000 people detained but by 1890 this figure had increased to over 86 000. If the increase in population from 16 million to 29 million is taken into account over this period, and the numbers of detained people is examined as a rate per 10 000 of the general population the results show a marked increase in the number of people officially detained as mad. Scull produces evidence from official figures which shows that, in 1844, for every 10 000 people there were 12.66 detained lunatics. However, by 1890 with the introduction of compulsory certification, this rate per 10 000 had risen to 29.26.

These statistics are only part of the story, as the largest single group within the detained population was the 'pauper lunatics'. As the asylums grew in number and scale during the second half of the nineteenth century, so did the number of pauper lunatics. This in itself would not be so remarkable if it were not for the evidence and arguments of the Poor Law Board. Their annual reports showed that the total numbers of paupers in England and Wales actually *decreased* during the second half of the century. At the same time the number of people classified and detained in the asylums as pauper lunatics increased. This development is partly explained by the establishment of better recording of statistics by local government, and the success of reformers in persuading parliament to ensure that each county made local provision for its own people. There are two other factors, however, which may go some way towards understanding these developments. Firstly, as the asylums were established as an alternative to the workhouse and the prison there was a pressing financial need to use the new asylums to the full. Secondly, the workhouse and the prison were already used by the parish and the magistrates, but the appearance of the asylum provided another alternative to dispose of people who were troubled or troublesome.

## THE UNINTENDED CONSEQUENCES OF REFORM

The change in provision for the mentally ill in the nineteenth century was more than just an increase in the number of asylums and beds available. A significant shift took place in the way in which society regarded lunacy and the lunatic. At the beginning of the nineteenth century the madhouses were feared as places of cruelty and neglect. By the end of the nineteenth century the fear of the asylum was no longer to do with cruelty. The dominant fear felt at all levels in society was concerned with the risk of wrongful detention in the public asylum. By the early part of the twentieth century public anxiety had changed again to add the fear of stigma associated with mental illness to the dread of certification and detention in the asylum. Within a century of the 1845 programme of reform which led to the compulsory building of the asylums, the long-standing fear of madness had been broadened to link social stigma with mental illness and mental illness services. The legacy of the nineteenth century asylums, which became synonymous with the treatment of mental illness was, in turn, to become the focus of efforts to change mental health policy, practice and provision. Ironically the evidence set out above shows that the majority of the asylum population were detained for economic circumstances rather than for clinical reasons.

The idea that policies directed at people with mental illness result from the dominant economic and political forces in society rather than from a medical view, has been explored by Foucault (1967) in his study of the treatment of mental illness during the French revolution. Scull (1975) looked at the way in which the idea of madness changed in Europe as society changed the ways in which it was organized and people earned their living. Warner (1985) took a similar materialist view of social change and compared differing cultures in order to look at the relationship between types of society and mental illness. Butler (1985) argued that the asylums became alternative places of disposal to the prisons and the workhouses for the magistrates who administered the system. The laws introduced at the end of the nineteenth century were intended to protect individuals from wrongful detention. In practice, however, the period after the passing of the Lunacy Act in 1890 led to an unprecedented *net* increase in the number of detained patients. One of the unintended consequences of these laws was to further isolate the mentally disordered and set them apart from society. This took place in two distinct ways. First, through the admission procedure which ensured that the only way to gain admission to the hospitals was through the use of compulsory legal detention using the 'certification' process. Second, with the use of the lunatic asylum as the most common way to detain and dispose of those admitted under the new lunacy law. This set the scene for much of the development of mental health policies up to the current period. For the 40 years following the introduction of the lunacy law up to the 1930s, the principal concerns of those working in mental health services was to find ways to overcome both the fear of certification and the social disgrace of the stigma associated with mental illness.

For those who followed on after the Second World War the agenda was set by the need to overcome much of the nineteenth century legacy and its consequences. In particular the three principal issues of admission without detention, hospital care without institutionalization, and care without stigma, dominated much of the official thinking on how mental health services were to be organized and delivered.

## PRESSURES FOR REFORM

Despite what has been said above it is important that we do not adopt attitudes of moral superiority toward those who set up and ran the asylums. This would only serve to cloud our judgements rather than to help to understand the real problems being confronted daily by policy-makers and practitioners. The nineteenth century pressure for the reform of the treatment of the mentally ill grew out of a reaction to the unacceptable quality of life provided in the private madhouses. In particular the birth of a reform movement to change the provision for the mentally ill was as a direct result of the scandals associated with the way in which people were admitted to, and detained in, the private madhouses.

The emergence of a reform movement, the passing of the lunacy laws and the creation of the public asylums was much more than a group of well-meaning individuals championing the plight of a group of people who were disadvantaged. Those individuals who lead the movement to reform policy and provision for people with mental illness were well meaning and the mentally ill were disadvantaged. However as a way of understanding the complex range of interrelated professional, political, economic and social issues this is not adequate explanation. The reform of the provision for the mentally ill was a rich amalgam of at least four differing pressures which eventually lead to the creation of the lunacy laws and the asylums.

It is worth taking a little time to explore and understand the pressures for reform and their consequences of patients and practitioners. The reform movement was successful in that it created a national approach to the mentally ill through the use of the public asylums. However, it also succeeded in producing some unintended consequences which have been set out above. To understand the importance of the achievements of the reform movement and their unintended consequences it is necessary to look separately in turn at the four pressures for change and to see what the practical outcomes were for the mentally ill and for those responsible for making policy and providing services.

Any reader looking at explanations of the past should try to understand the real problems confronting those who managed services and the ways in which they responded to them. In taking this view we may develop a more critical way of looking at our own policies and practices. The four pressures for change were a rich mixture of pressing practical problems and a new opportunity to introduce radical reform in society. In this sense the way in which society provided for the mentally ill was just one small example of wider changes which were to change economic life, social policy and the role of government. The four

key pressures are often treated in the literature on the emergence of mental illness social policy as if the issue had nothing
to do with politics and economics. They were as follows:

1.  **The impact of the market economy.** The first of the four
    pressures arose from fundamental changes in society and
    the way in which people earned their living. For centuries
    life was organized around village communities who cared
    for their own people through informal care arranged
    by the magistrate, the church and the poor law authorities.
    By the eighteenth century fundamental changes were under
    way which included the commercial development of agri-
    culture, the growth of industrial towns and the creation of
    a labour market. These changes had significant conse-
    quences for the mentally ill. Whilst it is important that we
    do not look at earlier practices uncritically, there is a need
    to grasp the significance of the changes brought about by
    the decline of the parish as the main way to provide for
    the mentally ill. What existed before the county asylum was
    essentially an informal approach to care which empha-
    sized local discretion and provision. This meant that the
    quality of care was dependent upon the judgments of local
    officials. However with such a system there was inevit-
    ably enormous variation in the range of provision. The type
    and quality of services available depended on where a
    person lived and, in this sense, whether a mentally ill per-
    son was treated well or badly was dependant or whether
    that person's parish provided for its poor and disturbed or
    did not.

2.  **Scandals and mistreatment.** Much of the time of the
    reformers was spent in investigating reported examples
    of cruelty and neglect which made up much of the report-
    ing of the plight of the mentally ill in the eighteenth and
    nineteenth century. For many people, provision for the
    mentally ill was associated with the fear of physical cruelty
    and neglect. The reformers spent much of their time
    involved in investigations and Royal Commissions looking
    at the circumstances of lunatics. Ironically much of the
    funding for the private madhouses came from the parish
    officials who were responsible for the administration of
    the poor law. The people who were provided for were

those regarded as the disturbed and the destitute. Therefore the private establishments increasingly were funded by monies from the public purse, despite a rising tide of unease concerning the experience of those housed in these places.

3. **The relationship between the individual and society.** This issue sounds superficially like a very abstract and obscure idea but it is one of the major concerns of politics. It was important in the campaign for the establishment of a parliamentary democracy in the 1820s and it still applies to the central questions of government policies in the 1990s. At its heart is the quesiton as to how much the state should intervene in the business of individuals to limit, constrain or control their behaviour. In the case of a person who is said to be mentally ill the issue is to do with the degree to which an individual's behaviour is the responsibility of that person alone. What is also asked is at what point society, through the state, should set limits and take action to prevent an individual doing as he liked. Such a question was all the more relevant in the world of the nineteenth century where the right of the individual was being asserted through trade and industry. The new economic doctrines of capitalism were to transform the way in which traditional society operated. For those people who were unable to labour and fend for themselves it was important in such a world that a balance was achieved between social duty and economic beliefs. In practice there was a long-standing acceptance of the role of the parish to take social responsibility for the destitute, whilst discouraging dependency and indolence. Therefore there emerged a series of policies which emphasized the use of the feared institution as way of providing for a range of dependant groups as a matter of the last resort. It was soon realized that if the institutions were large enough that it would be possible to make places available at a much lower cost than in the small private madhouses.

4. **The idea that public institutions could be well managed.** Underpinning this approach was the idea that it was possible to establish 'good government' which was based on the sound principles of industry and create an economic way of providing for those people who were unable to

earn their own living. The move towards a new system
of public care based on the institution arose out of the need
to establish an alternative to the private madhouses.
However the task facing the reformers was more complicated than this. As well as creating an alternative to
mistreatment they had to make the case for a cost-effective
service and show that the new system was better than the
one it replaced. In responding to this challenge the
reformers looked to their own experience and from this
they developed proposals for a new way to administer the
asylums. At the heart of these proposals was the idea that
inspection would play a vital role in the surveillance of the
mentally ill and the asylums. The reformers argued for the
creation of an independent inspectorate to visit asylums
and madhouses regularly and report annually to parliament on the state of the public and private madhouses.
Many of those involved in the reform movement believed
that the campaign for reform of the arrangements for the
lunatics was part of a wider reform movement for the creation of good government. By 'good government' the
reformers meant not only the way that it was elected and
claimed to be representative, but also the quality of the
services provided by both central and local government.

ENDURING RELATIONSHIPS FOR THE MENTALLY ILL

The reformers argued that the answer to the abuses of the
private madhouses was to create an alternative system of
provision for the mentally disturbed. In this sense the approach
taken to the mentally ill proved to be an early example of a
general approach towards dealing with troubled and troublesome groups in society. The approach developed towards the
mentally ill in the middle of the nineteenth century had two
remarkable properties. First, it proved to be robust in that it
has persisted to the present day. Second, the three key relationships established 150 years ago have shaped many of our
policies and practices today. To understand the significance
of the influence of earlier policies we need to look more closely
in turn at the three persistent themes referred to at the beginning of this chapter. In particular we need to understand the
form in which this Victorian legacy presents itself today.

1.  **The continued use of Victorian hospitals.** For the majority of patients who receive mental health services in Britain, even when services are provided in the community they are characterized in relation to the hospital. The whole experience is based on the relationship of institutional care provided in the hospital with the individual patient. Services are described in terms of 'acute', 'chronic' or 'after-care'. The focus of the relationship between provider and recipient of service remains the institution, the hospital. The asylums created in the nineteenth century which have become our old mental hospitals persist as the dilapidated homes for many elderly patients. In contrast to the physical decline of the buildings the negative image of mental illness and the mentally ill is reinforced daily as a powerful and potent reminder to the rest of society.

2.  **The stereotype of the person with mental illness as being pitiful or dangerous.** This idea persists at the root of our legislation. Social policy for the mentally ill continues to include the use of compulsory legal powers to detain, admit and treat patients. The consequences of this approach can be far-reaching for the future quality of life for patients as it can lead to social stigma, bewilderment and a sense of personal powerlessness. This is despite the fact that compulsory detention is used for a small minority of patients in hospital and for an even smaller proportion of those people who use mental health services.

3.  **Compulsory detention of people with mental illness.** The success of the reform movement was the creation of the public asylums, lead by doctors who claimed to be the new experts in lunacy along with the fledgling nursing profession which manned the wards and in time replaced the old workhouse turnkeys. Their activities were inspected by the new Commissioners in Lunacy who visited and produced annual reports. Admission was made through the magistrate who acted in response to applications from the parish Relieving Officer of the Poor. Today mental health services are usually delivered through psychiatric services led by doctors and supported by nurses. Annual inspections are made by the Mental Health Act commissioners concerned with the minority of detained patients whose application for admission is often made by the local authority social worker.

In some respects so much has changed since the end of the nineteenth century, but in many ways little has changed as the powerful legacy of the past continues to influence current roles, policy and practices.

What resulted from these forces and pressures was a system which was regarded as humane and progressive which mirrored a society which took its responsibilities seriously towards the less fortunate. For us the significance of these developments is not so much their historical interest but rather the way in which they continue to impact on current services. The professional relationships described above have largely persisted to the present day for most of mental health care. The relationship between the doctor, nurse, social worker and Mental Health Act Commissioner can be recognized from their counterparts in the nineteenth century asylum.

## ALTERNATIVES TO THE ASYLUM

There are two further points to be made in this opening chapter which are important to our understanding of the development of policies and practices for the care of the mentally ill. The first of these is to do with the form of care offered to the mentally ill. The second is to do with the political issues which became tied up with the rights of the individual and the use of the asylum.

The question of the models of care used in the institutions is not as straightforward as it might first appear. As there was nothing inevitable about the creation of the large asylums. The task of investigating cruel treatment and the emergence of an alternative approach to the care of the mentally ill was hard won. However, it was not inevitable that a large asylum would be run as a self-sufficient enterprise like a great factory; there were alternative systems available. Prominent amongst the reform movement was William Tuke who has already been mentioned for his work in investigations and the notion of 'moral treatment' as an alternative to physical restraint. This approach was concerned with the use of small, family-type institutions to care for the mentally ill where the patient was well-treated and cared for in a quasi-religious community. Some of the work of Tuke and his family at 'The Retreat' in York is partially similar to the later approaches taken by the therapeutic communities. But Tuke and his approach was not the only alternative to mistreatment in the asylums or madhouses. Even within the large public asylums there were attempts made to develop an alternative to the physical control of the residents. Prominent in what became known as the 'non-restraint' movement were practising doctors in the asylums such as John Conolly, who worked at the Hanwell asylum in the late 1840s. However, with the large number of asylum patients from the middle of the century, there proved to be few followers of the alternatives to the large institutions which used physical restraint.

As well as the question of differing or preferred models of care there was also a political dimension to the reform of the lunacy policies in the nineteenth century. The first of these was the growing belief in the role of the economic market in regulating many aspects of life. The second was the idea that it was possible to establish good government on the lines of science and enterprise. What resulted from these two beliefs is one of the key developments of British politics of the nineteenth century. There appeared a society which was increasingly confident of the ability of the market to solve and regulate most of human behaviour at the same time as the case was being made for the idea of humane and scientific government. These two conflicting beliefs, of the non-interfering government and the successful centralized state has persisted in British politics to the present day. The recurring impact of these two conflicting ideas will be explored in later chapters of this book.

For people with mental illness the position by the end of the nineteenth century was paradoxical. The reform campaign to overcome the misuse of the madhouses had led to the struggle for the creation of the public asylums. By 1890, however, when the lunacy laws were introduced, there was a widespread public fear of being wrongfully detained in the new asylums. But the new law did far more than just distinguish between those who needed to be certified and those who did not. The legal route to asylum admission was determined not by medical condition but by economic status. The Lunacy Act 1890 provided for four forms of admission: of these, reception, urgency and inquisition orders required medical recommendations and applied only to private patients. There was a separate certification for 'pauper lunatics' who had to go through a judicial procedure before being admitted to the asylum on summary reception orders. The majority of the asylum population were 'pauper lunatics' admitted by the use of summary reception orders. This involved the Poor Law Relieving Officer, a Justice of the Peace and two medical practitioners to complete an order. For those people found wandering a constable could initially admit to the workhouse.

What is significant about the arrangements for the mentally ill by 1890 is that the patients were classified not by either medical condition or behaviour but by **socio-economic status**. Separate legal and administrative procedures were established for the majority of those people detained: the pauper lunatics. What began as a campaign against cruel treatment ended as a series of measures to protect citizens against wrongful detention in the asylum. What is so remarkable about the situation by 1890 is the virtual absence of any references to treatment which had so preoccupied the reform movement for the preceding half century. It was this issue of access to treatment and the fear and social stigma of certification associated with the admission to the asylum which was to shape subsequent attempts to reform mental health policy and practice.

What we need to understand is that those people who fought and argued for the creation of the asylums did so in the belief that they were doing good to those less fortunate than themselves. In the name of doing good there arose a system of providing for people with mental illness which cut them off from mainstream society and rendered them powerless. This view of the past is intended to act as a warning against complacency, as our policies and practices may well be looked on with loathing and puzzlement by practitioners and service-users in the future.

# 2

# From custody to therapy

ORDINARY LIVES?: PATIENTS AND STAFF
IN THE OLD HOSPITALS

The words we use to describe the social world around us
change their meaning over time to such a degree that they can
become barely recognizable to those who first used them. This
is often the case with health and welfare services as the word
'care' and especially 'community care' is often used in such
a way that it virtually looses all real meaning. The word 'care'
can be used as a verb to talk of being concerned, to worry,
to disapprove, to care for and to tend. As a noun it reads as
trouble, prudence, regarding and being anxious. Such a simple
word is loaded with meaning when used in specific social
context such as being 'in care' or 'receiving care' in the
community.

In the same way the word 'asylum' is simultaneously full
of meaning and quite empty. Today it is more often used as
a term of abuse or failure rather than as a word to describe
accurately a form of provision. The use of the term to refer
to a 'haven', 'refuge', 'retreat', 'shelter' or 'sanctuary' has
almost passed from common use. To talk of asylum for people
with mental illness increasingly divides the speaker and the
listener as being on opposite sides of the institution versus
community divide. This is all the more confusing as the word
asylum was used in the early and middle parts of the nineteenth century to signify a new form of provision run along
humane and rational lines. By the end of the nineteenth
century the asylum had become a place for the disposal of those
who were certified. Like the workhouse it was feared by

those who were admitted to it and largely ignored by those who lived in the towns and cities around which the institutions were clustered. For other peole the asylums were places of work and for those detained as patients they all too often became 'home'.

This chapter will look at life in the asylums for both patients and staff and the changes in provision for the mentally ill, which were to prove to be a challenge to the old hospitals. In particular the changing perceptions of the role of the asylums will be examined, along with the attempts to establish therapeutic approaches to patient care. This is particularly important as 'therapy' is often regarded uncritically as both desirable and necessary, without understanding the range of approaches it can include or their implications for the service-user. A starting point for understanding the change in approach to patients and their treatment is to examine the capacity of the asylums to endure external changes in society at large and internally within the institutions themselves.

At the very time that the lunacy laws were being enacted in the last decade of the nineteenth century, the movement towards an alternative approach to the care of the mentally ill was taking root. This lead to a situation which was paradoxical in that mental disorder was seen as part of a disease process which needed medical care provided by the specialist doctors in the asylums. However the introduction of certification brought with it the twin stigmas of loss of liberty and confinement in the asylum as well as a label of lunatic. For the majority of those detained in the institutions the asylum was an alternative to the workhouse or casual vagrancy. The asylums were, in effect, self-sufficient communities on the margins of the great towns and cities where the material needs of the resident population were provided. The asylums provided shelter, sanctuary, food and recreation for the detained. For those who were capable of work there was a life of domestic or agricultural work to provide for others in the institution.

Like their patients the professional staff in the asylums were based in the institutions and to a lesser degree shared some of the stigma of the people they cared for and controlled. The idea that the mental medicine practiced in the asylum could do more than care, control and detain would have been viewed with scepticism by professionals and public alike. Ironically, it had been demonstrated that the earlier approach of moral management had produced improved functioning for patients without the use of doctors or a medical explanation of the patients' problems. It is clear that the asylums played a wider role than as a place for medical practice. The asylum served at times as a means of direct social control, a refuge and as a concerted way to study madness.

As has already been shown in Chapter 1, the majority of the nineteenth century residents in the asylum were there for economic rather than medical reasons. In coming to terms with the nineteenth century legacy for mental health services it is important to understand that the population which lived in the asylums of the last century is in many ways distinctly different from the mental hospital populations of the late twentieth century. This theme will be followed up in more detail in Chapter 3. As a preface to this discussion we need to have a better understanding of the quality of life offered by the nineteenth century asylum and the ways in which mental health services were marginalized within the other professions. In particular, we need to grasp the implications of these developments for the emergence of new health and social care policy and practice in the twentieth century.

## QUALITY OF LIFE IN THE ASYLUM

The asylums were large in scale where resident populations of over 2000 were not uncommon. In such settings there developed a number of contradictory strands. To the local economy the asylum became a significant employer. In the new occupation of nursing which arose out of the old turnkey function of the prison and the madhouse, there emerged a respectable and relatively secure type of employment. Whereas the weekly wage was low there was a high degree of security and personal power within the confines of the asylum. It became a characteristic of the larger asylums for there to be a number of generations of the same family employed in the institutions. In this sense they were to become alternatives to the fields and the factories for numbers of workers. Despite the economic importance to the local economy the institutions were often represented as places of fear and danger.

In contrast to this popular image the daily life in asylums was often one of drudgery and tedium. The asylum was a place of confinement, not a centre for medical practice. However out of the asylums there grew the speciality of mental medicine which in turn became psychiatry. The life of the resident patient was governed by the rhythms of the large institutions which reduced the complexity of individual preferences and needs to a repeatable and economic formula to which all conformed. All activities were strictly completed by rote at the prescribed times including eating, recreation and work. The role of the resident patient was not to take part in a therapeutic regimen, as such a function did not exist. Rather, the role of the patient was essentially twofold: first, to be an accepting inmate of the asylum; second, to be a casual labourer in one of the institution's self-sufficent enterprises. The asylum did provide a refuge from the harsh realities of the growing industrial world outside, but at a significant personal cost to the residents. This cost included the loss of liberty, the acceptance of a social stigma, emotional and cultural poverty as well as the grinding routine of a life totally regulated by the needs of the institution itself. In return the asylum provided the necessities of life which perhaps were only available through the workhouse or petty crime for those who were unable to labour.

For those who worked in the large institutions the asylum provided a mixture of blessings. Initially, for the medical profession which provided the leadership to the institution, there was the recognition that they held a special position of authority; increasingly there was the shared belief that the doctors were the experts in mental medicine. This brought with it a number of consequences. Within the asylum it brought a position of power and influence whereas within the profession of medicine it brought a sense of isolation from the physicians and surgeons. One common feature of nurses and doctors in the asylum was the way in which they used their place in the institutions to pursue greater professional status. Where else but within a closed community such as an asylum, was it better to develop specialist knowledge of a group of people who were regarded by society with a mixture of fear, loathing and pity.

By the early part of this century there were significant developments in the organization of the asylum workforce. Nurses and hospital Almoners had created representative bodies in general medicine just after the turn of the century; by 1910 the asylum workers had established their own trades union. The express purpose of the new unions was to improve the working conditions and rewards of ancillary staff within the asylums. Medical staff working within the asylums had also begun to organize themselves effectively. As early as 1848 the asylum doctors had founded the *Journal of Psychological Medicine* and *Mental Pathology* and by 1853 they had established their own *Asylum Journal*. By 1911, the year after the founding of the Asylum Workers Union the first professional qualification specifically for work with the mentally ill was established. The Diploma in Psychological Medicine was introduced with the assistance of the universities and the Royal Colleges. This development was significant in three key respects. First, it brought mental medicine closer professionally to the long-established physicians and surgeons. Second, it gave the disparate group of medical practitioners in the isolated asylums a common network which enabled them to negotiate collectively. Third, it served to set apart those who possessed expert knowledge of the state of mind of the mentally ill from the rest of the population. In short, the earlier claims of the asylum doctors to have specialist insight into the world of the mentally ill was matched institutionally by the introduction of formal academic qualifications.

For the patients and residents of the asylums there were no collective organizations of their own to represent their views, aspirations and needs. However, there were a number of voluntary organizations specifically to provide assistance to patients after discharge from the large asylums. These aftercare associations were created in the last two decades of the nineteenth century and, although modest in ambition, they did at least look to the possibility of life outside the asylum for the mentally ill. Despite this, the focus of patient care remained the asylum itself; the professionalization of the asylum workforce further emphasized that the institution was the place for the care of the mentally ill.

## THE RISE OF THERAPY

Shortly after the introduction of the lunacy laws at the end of the nineteenth century a slow process of change began to take root which was to challenge much of official thinking on the provision for the mentally ill. This process did not arise from a single issue or development: three different developments resulted in the first stirrings of change in government thinking – away from the legal provision of asylums to incarcerate certified lunatics. The first development was a series of investigations on public health which highlighted the relationship between poor health and poverty. The second notion which was gaining ground was that it was not only possible but desirable to provide care for people with mental illness without certification. The third strand in this process was the acceptance that mental disorder was a form of illness, treatable by medicine, and that new treatments could be developed for mental illness as in other branches of medicine. Between them these changes opened the way for a limited but innovative range of therapies which could not only explain but also treat mental illness. This type of therapeutic optimism was to prove to be a frustrated feature of many new practices in the mental health field. The process which began before the First World War was to continue until the beginning of the 1960s.

It will be argued in Chapter 3 that the rise of therapy or a range of therapies was not a liberation for patients as it owed more to professional rivalry between competing explanations of the causes and treatment of mental illness. It will also be argued that many basic civil rights have yet to be won for patients including their right to have access to services that they choose to engage with. However, to understand the origins of the present position it is necessary to look first in some detail at the three interwoven strands referred to above.

## HEALTH, MEDICINE AND GOVERNMENT

The new role established by central government in the nineteenth century included an investigative arm through the use of official enquiries including Royal Commissions which reported directly to parliament. From the turn of the twentieth century these committees were active in looking at social issues, especially those concerned with social deprivation, health and welfare. The attraction of the Royal Commissions was twofold to both government and the parliamentarians. First, they ensured that pressing social issues were aired in a non-party-political way and second, they paved the way for legislation without rushing through reforms. Royal Commissions which referred to the plight of the mentally ill appeared shortly after the turn of the century. By the end of the first decade of the century there were official reports on physical health, 'feeble-mindedness' and the Poor Law. The report of 1909 called for the abolition of the Poor Law administration and the introduction of national assistance income maintenance for the poor. Despite the fact that the Commission made majority and minority reports there was agreement on the need to reduce the harm and fear associated with the Poor Laws. Despite this report it was to take another 40 years to see out the influence of the Poor Law with the introduction of the Welfare State.

The Commissioners in Lunacy were replaced in 1913 by the Board of Control which continued the role of inspection and annual reporting to parliament established in the middle of the nineteenth century which was referred to in Chapter 1. These changes were part of a set of legal reforms which brought a new approach to the care of the mentally handicapped which was symbolized by the change in terms from the care of the 'feeble-minded' to services for the 'mentally deficient'. The significance of the legislation was that it distinguished between mental illness and mental handicap and it officially recognized that the asylum was not the only venue for work in the mental health field.

Reference has already been made in Chapter 1 to the range of approaches to the treatment of the mentally ill in the nineteenth century. They varied from traditional informal care in the villages to admission to the asylum. Although the use of certification in the public asylum became the main strategy of public policy for the mentally ill, there were other parallel approaches developed in the nineteenth century. Moral treatment and the non-restraint movement has already been discussed, as has the rise of asylum medicine. By the turn of the twentieth century a number of other approaches to mental illness were being developed. A number of institutions referred to themselves as 'Mental hospitals' and by 1907 the London County Council was negotiating with Dr Henry Maudsley who was keen to fund and open a mental hospital specifically to allow for early treatment for the mentally ill. Maudsley was a rather unlikely figure to propose such a move as he was a major figure of the medical establishment, working in the asylums in the late nineteenth century. However, he was also the son-in-law of Dr John Conolly of Hanwell who had pioneered the use of non-restraint in the first half of the nineteenth century. The Maudsley Hospital was opened in 1915 with a remit to ensure that patients received early treatment, in contrast to the asylums which continued to emphasize detention and loss of liberty.

Following the alliance described above between local government, voluntary organizations and health professionals the rise of a therapeutic approach had begun in earnest. This resulted in easier access to mental health services without the disruption and stigma of mental hospital admission. The irony of this situation should not be lost, as much of the second half of this century has been spent in trying to ensure that health and local authority services are not fragmented for patients and clients. In a number of local developments it was demonstrated that coherent and integrated services can be provided if there is a common vision and a flexibility in the way services are organized. This is an issue which has dogged much of social policy in the mental health field and which forms the core problem of community care services which is the subject of Chapter 3. The developments of the 1930s did more than nurture new approaches to mental health practice as once again they highlighted significant inequalities in the availability of mental health services. As before, the key factor in gaining access to the new approaches was economic status rather than health and social need.

The First World War also provided a significant challenge for the asylums and the services available for the mentally ill. Moreover the period from 1914 to 1918 lead to a questioning of the nature of mental illness itself and the range of psychological problems experienced by military personnel. Some of the inconsistencies in official thinking became more apparent as health and welfare agencies had to deal with soldiers who were psychologically disturbed by their war experience, either through their own injuries or the experience of war. It proved to be difficult to sustain the view that those who suffered from mental illness were prone to it as a consequence of poor breeding when they had already proved themselves in combat and were regarded as national heroes. Whereas the First World War was to challenge some of the preconceptions regarding the mentally ill held by social policy-makers, the Second World War was to influence official thinking on the usefulness of psychiatric and psychological services.

Official reports and enquiries continued throughout the 1920s and 1930s and these lead to changes in the organization of health and welfare provision. In 1919 a Ministry of Health was created which brought together the Local Government Board, the Insurance Commissioners, the Public Health section of the Privy Council, the Board of Education and the Home Office Department for Mental Diseases. By 1920 the Board of Control was transferred to the new Ministry of Health and the idea that mental disorder was an illness received official approval at government level. Following a widely publicized court case concerning the treatment of a patient in a private asylum, and a book by Dr Lomax (1924) which accused Prestwich Hospital in Lancashire of poor conditions and illegal detention, there followed a period of parliamentary discussion on the provision for the mentally ill. Dr Lomax had also called into question the developing role of psychiatry and this had provoked a debate within the medical profession. The Minister of Health responded by establishing a Royal Commission in 1924 which reported in 1926. This report lead directly to the Mental Treatment Act of 1930 which introduced significant changes as it emphasized the place of professional discretion, judgement and decision-making rather than certification. The act continued to allow for compulsory admission as well as two new categories of patients who were admitted on either a voluntary basis or for temporary hospital care. The slow corrosion of the approach established by the Victorian lunacy laws had begun. The 1930s legislation gave greater authority to the doctors who worked in mental medicine and changed the local authority official from the nineteenth century role of 'Relieving Officer of the Poor' to the 'Duly Authorised Officer'. This title was to persist as the legal name for the social worker until 1959 when it became the 'Mental Welfare Officer'. Moreover, the 1930s legislation allowed for the first time for patients to be treated in public hospitals without having to be subject to the stigma associated with the Victorian lunacy laws or to undergo certification. The idea of early informal treatment had been accepted officially and provided for in a limited way in the legislation on mental illness. The very title of the act referred to 'treatment' which was indicative of the degree to which the rise of therapy was evident, albeit haltingly and unevenly.

As mental health policy changed in the 1930s with the easing of admission procedures to hospitals and there was an emerging expectation that a more treatment-oriented approach should be developed; so the long, slow decline of the old asylums began. The starting point for this process was the completion of the building programme which meant that there was to be little new capital investment in the mental hospitals. Over the following 50 years the physical state of the buildings was to decline as the population aged with it. Eventually this was to lead to a challenge to the idea that hospitals were the only and most appropriate place to treat mental illness and in turn this led to a government programme for resettlement and closure. However, between the therapeutic optimism for the 1930s legislation and a more comprehensive policy on mental health care, there was a period of 15 years of activity, change and development in health and social care which was to shape much of subsequent development.

Undoubtedly the Second World War made a significant impact on the future of mental health policy and provision but not in a way that was predictable or obvious. During the 1939–1945 period, three separate strands became tightly interwoven in a way which was to influence the future of mental health policy and practice. The first and most significant of these strands was the campaign for the creation of a National Health Service, free at the point of delivery as an alternative to the pre-war arrangement of 'private' and 'panel' patients which resulted in major regional inequalities in health. This development not only changed the way in which health care was organized and provided, it also radically changed the role of government in giving new civil rights to all citizens.

The second of the three strands was the practical effect of the war emergency on the stock of resources available to mental health services. At the outbreak of war, large numbers of asylums were taken over wholesale and transformed into medical, surgical and convalescent units for the armed forces and injured civilians, thereby reducing the numbers of beds available for mental patients. This development had two key impacts: first, it led to the rapid discharge of some patients who did not return to the asylums and, second, it led to the widespread understanding within the health professions that alternative methods of treatment would have to be established which did not rely on long-stay hospital care for the mentally ill.

The third strand in this argument is the changed perception of the standing of psychiatrists in official thinking. At the beginning of the war much of mental health care including the psychiatrists was marginal to modern health and social care. As a result of their use in the armed forces during the war, albeit in personnel selection, the psychiatrists gained greatly in professional standing. The old claim to be the experts in madness was true only in the context of the isolated asylums, but by 1945 there was widespread acceptance that the psychiatrist was the expert in mental illness. The challenge facing them by 1945 was to demonstrate this in terms of the efficacy of their practice. Before that challenge can be examined it is important to look at the creation of the National Health Service and its implications for people with mental illness.

## THE NATIONAL HEALTH SERVICE: UNFULFILLED PROMISES FOR THE MENTALLY ILL

Before the Second World War there was an active, public, political campaign for the provision of health services free at the point of delivery. Much of the argument was tied up with the idea of citizenship and health and welfare services as a civil right. Whilst there were many voices from the left calling for such provision there was also a growing political consensus which sought the creation of a health system. This was seen as an alternative to the three types of providers which existed: the voluntary and university hospitals, the small specialist centres and the Poor-Law infirmaries. These hospitals were just that, hospitals rather than health centres or services. The form of care offered was selective rather than universal and they produced a pattern of health care which generated and emphasized regional inequalities in health. In practice this meant that the quality of health care enjoyed by any individual or family was a function of both their social class and an accident of geography, as health care varied greatly from place to place. The war quickly lead to hospitals coming under central government control and in the context of a national emergency the arguments for and against the public control of health resources was set aside.

The detailed arguments concerning the creation of the National Health Service have been the focus of a number of studies, many of which concentrated on the political battle between the British Medical Association and the new Labour government of 1945. The vehicle for the creation of the National Health Service and what became the 'Welfare State' was the report by William Beveridge entitled 'Social Insurance and Allied Services' published in 1942. Beneath the dry and restrained title was shallowly hidden the means to achieve a set of social policy reforms which would largely remain unaltered for over 40 years.

The shape of the modern Welfare State was formed by the war-time experience of the national emergency. As a direct consequence of the campaign to win the war through military means, there arose a struggle to win the peace through new social policies. The testing ground for these new approaches was to be the parliamentary ballot box. By 1945 the hundreds of thousands of returning military forces had developed an expectation that having won the war they would now benefit from the peace. The Beveridge proposals caught this mood accurately in that it addressed two of the key social policies by suggesting wholesale changes in health provision and income maintenance. In place of the fragmented and uneven hospital service it was proposed that a National Health Service should be established free at the point of delivery. In place of the feared Poor-Law arrangements it was proposed to establish a system of national assistance to ensure a basic adequate income for all. These new services were to be paid for by taxation and national insurance; whilst they were free at the point of delivery they were not free *per se*, as they were funded from the salaries and wages of the working population.

The proposals of 1942 became part of the electoral battle of 1945 when the national government lead by the Conservative war Prime Minister Winston Churchill was replaced by a Labour administration headed by Clement Attlee. The parliamentary sessions of 1946 and 1947 were dominated by discussions of the future developments of health and welfare provision. The result of these deliberations was the founding of the Welfare State through the National Health Services Act 1946 and the National Assistance Act 1948. These two pieces of legislation came into force in 1948, by which time other signifi-cant changes were under way in social provision, including education and housing. The arguments developed in the 1920s and 1930s setting out the cases for a national health system pointed to the shortcomings of the old system, especially in the regional differences it produced in health care. By the 1940s there was a growing belief that the mentally ill were additionally disadvantaged as some of their needs were clinical whilst others were social. Therefore any system of health and welfare provi-sion which was likely to be adequate to meet the needs of the mentally ill would have to be integrated into a single approach.

In reality, the lack of an integrated approach to the needs of the mentally ill persisted throughout the reforms of the late 1940s and continues to the present day as a fundamental obstacle to coherent services for the mentally ill. It is necessary to look at the detail of provision for the mentally ill at the time of the creation of the welfare state, in order to understand the current preoccupation with community care policies and the respective positions of the health service and local authority social services. It will be argued here that the roots of many problems faced by contemporary services are to be found in the arrangements made in 1948 and after. For the mentally ill this lead to fragmented services and missed opportunities.

The idea that services for the mentally ill should be integrated into the rest of a National Health Service gained ground during the war. The *British Medical Journal* argued in editorials in 1943 for psychiatry to be based in, and practised within, local general hospitals as part of an integrated health service. This idea was to reoccur as a feature of government policy in the 1970s as it looked for ways to reform provision for the mentally ill. The detail of this policy and the consequences it had for those working in mental health services will be discussed in Chapter 3.

## FRAGMENTED MENTAL HEALTH SERVICES

The new health service of 1948 was based on an organizational principal of integration through the use of local health centres which would act as the social cement between the hospital service, general practitioners and local authority welfare services. The National Health Service began life on the 'appointed day', the 5th July 1948, and brought with it almost half a million hospital beds in over 2500 separate hospitals. These hospital services were managed by new Area Health Authorities which administered local services on behalf of the Ministry of Health. Despite the fact that almost half the total number of beds in the new service were for the mentally ill they appear as marginal to the mainstream discussions of the period. Mental illness and the mentally ill figure little in the official annual reports of the Ministry of Health in the period immediately after the creation of the National Health Service, despite the belief that they were integral parts of the new arrangements.

Despite the principle of integrated services the legislation which introduced the Welfare State actively worked against the possibilities of a coherent services for the mentally ill. The National Assistance Act, 1948, brought an end to the Poor Law. This was widely welcomed as the old act both failed to provide adequately and stigmatized those who received relief. For most people, the Poor Law and the workhouses were one and the same. However the National Assistance Act gave to the local authority a **power** to provide services but it did not make it a **duty**. This meant that it was at the discretion of each local authority as to whether they provided particular services. In practice this meant that whether or not a person received welfare services was dependent on where they lived. Whereas one authority might provide a range of services for those residents with a mental health problem, a neighbouring authority might not provide any such service. The situation by 1948 was heavy with irony for those who worked in the mental health field and especially so for those who received services. The Welfare State had heralded the introduction of a new approach to health and income maintenance services which was national. In principal the service should be the same irrespective of the home address of the patient or recipient of benefit. In practice, however, the requirement to meet the social needs of local authority clients was dependent on local policies, politics and resources.

The most visible sign of the changes in welfare provision was in the care of the elderly with the demise of the workhouse and the introduction of residential homes run by the local authority. The mentally ill appear as half-forgotten silent partners in the policy changes of the late 1940s. The original impetus to the campaign for reform was the scandal of regional inequalities in health care. The new Welfare State of 1948 did little for the mentally ill directly; despite their significance numerically, they were a sideshow to the mainstream activity of developing the acute services of the new health authorities. The mentally ill and their social needs figure relatively little in the post-war world of social reconstruction, where building houses for the baby boom and providing education for growing children were the new priorities.

The debates on national social policy throughout the 1940s went to the heart of modern political beliefs in that the relationship between the individual and the state was re-examined. More particularly the arguments were concerned with the degree to which the state should intervene into the lives of individuals. The outcome of the debates was the modern Welfare State which has suffered more than most institutions from a careless use of language and poorly formulated descriptions of the role and function of health and welfare services.

Despite the much reported apolitical origins of the health and welfare reforms – commissioned by a Conservative Prime Minister, drafted by a Liberal administrator and introduced by a Labour government – a basic ambiguity persists as regards services provided. To the political right, welfare services provided for the minimum necessary intervention to enable an individual to live their life without interference. To the political left, welfare represented a civil right for all in the community to access comprehensive services to meet a range of social needs. The issue of rights and responsibilities goes to the heart of public policy and practice in the mental health field and appears as a recurrent theme in this book. The opposing beliefs of the political right and left is a form of convenient short-hand to summarize the debate on the role of the state and the degree to which it should be involved in the lives of individuals and communities. This point underpinned the discussion in Chapter 1 on the idea of good government and the role of properly managed public institutions in the nineteenth century. To the political right the question is posed in terms of rights as a 'freedom to' do things without interference, whereas to the left it is seen as a 'freedom from' want and need.

This debate may superficially appear to be arid and dry but it is applied in practical ways in public policy in the mental health field. The clearest examples are those to do with compliance to treatment and the way in which this is applied and enforced. If the orientation of a mental health service is towards hospital care then there is often an implied threat to rights through the use of compulsory detention. In a community setting the issue is no less applicable: for example, the way in which outreach work is established may be at the cost of the rights of the individual service-user if benefits money is only made available on a daily basis following attendance at a community centre. This issue of rights and responsibilities has developed clearly since the 1970s in American mental health care following the efforts to close the old hospitals and this will be discussed further in Chapter 7.

It is important to recognize that the origins of this debate can be found in the nineteenth century experience and it persists as a recurring issue for mental health professionals and users. During the mid to late 1940s, as the National Health Service (NHS) was being introduced, there was a renewed debate on the role of the state and government. It was veiled under the issue of protecting or challenging the traditional arrangements of hospital and health care provision. In the mental health field this issue was not to be resolved as quickly or easily. It will be argued later that much of the arguments and changes of the early 1990s are informed by the same set of unresolved and persistent issues in British public policy on health and social care.

As the NHS was being debated and planned there were some changes in the mental health field itself, not least in those hospitals who had experienced requisitioning of their facilities and the discharge of large numbers of patients in order to accommodate the physically injured returning from combat. At the same time there was an increasing interest in the development of day care for the mentally ill, but the infrastructure necessary to provide a range of therapeutic services simply did not exist. Most notable for their absence both within the mental hospitals and in day-care facilities were the psychiatric social workers. One of the characteristics of the social policy literature of the late 1940s and early 1950s is the emphasis on the lack of trained psychiatric social workers. It was also argued that access to this discipline would greatly increase the possibility of discharging a patient from a mental hospital. What is not said, all too often, is that local authorities failed to provide any recognizable form of mental health service, save for the duly authorized officer whose statutory duty was to make applications for compulsory admission to the mental hospital.

Rather than being surprised that mental health services were failing by the early 1950s, it would be much more puzzling if they were thriving, given the organizational obstacles to coherent service delivery. Central government set the social policy objectives and agendas and divided the tasks between departments of central and local govenrment. Some of these were duties which had to be provided as a statutory require-ment whilst others were powers which were or were not provided given the choice of individual departments. The issue of functions being split between agencies with a range of uncoordinated perspectives and responsibilities was to dog the policy and practice of mental health provision for the following 40 years. From the point of view of an individual service-user or carer, it must have seemed as if the whole system was designed to ensure that it was organizationally impossible to provide a comprehensive and coherent service to patients and clients. Four decades later all of those involved in health and social care would still be struggling with a problem which was built into the first phase of the Welfare State in 1948.

## 3

# Community care:
# the elusive solution

One of the most powerful beliefs in modern British social policy
is the idea that the 1950s saw a revolutionary transformation
in provision for the mentally ill. This is such a significant claim
that it needs to be examined in some detail; it has an important
bearing on the way in which we understand the recent
development of mental health services and the origins of
current policies and practices. It will be argued here that such
a claim is mythical and overplayed: for the majority of the
mentally ill the experience was isolating, stigmatizing and painful. The case for a revolution in the care of the mentally ill in
the 1950s is most clearly set out by Jones (1972). Jones argues
that there were three 'revolutions' in the treatment of the
mentally ill in the 1950s, in the approach to medical treatment,
admission policies and legal provision. Such a view is enormously appealing as it would make coherent a number of
separate developments and would provide a single framework
for understanding complex technical and policy changes.
However the evidence does not lend itself to such a neat
explanation.

The first of the three revolutions was in the way medical
practice developed, especially in the use of medication through
the introduction of psychotropic drugs. However the majority
of patients who were detained in the large old hospitals did
not enjoy the benefits of revolutionary new therapies. For them
it was the routine of daily institutional life which shaped

their experience rather than a new technology. What was underway by the middle of the 1950s was the emergence of a two-tier system of provision for the mentally ill which was to replace the nineteenth century public versus private distinction in lunacy. The new categories were that of chronic versus acute mental patient which allowed a dual system of care standards to develop. Only if such a dichotomy is ignored can it be argued that changes in medical practice were revolutionary.

The second of the three revolutions was said to be in the administrative changes which lead to the so-called 'open door' policy to enable easier access to services for the mentally ill. Jones argues that the ability to receive hospital treatment and care without detention or certification was a revolutionary change. What was actually involved was an expansion of the approach made possible by the Mental Treatment Act 1930, which provided access for some patients to voluntary admission. This avoided the use of both the lunacy laws and the stigma of the old asylums. However the benefits of open door access to the mental hospital need to be considered more carefully, especially in terms of the civil rights of individual patients and the treatments they received. By allowing informal access to services the patient was tacitly giving consent to treatment and therefore there was a significant transfer of personal power from the patient to the hospital providing the treatment. Clearly, for most patients this arrangement was likely to work well as staff worked professionally and acted honourably. Such a system was, however, based on a principal which could be abused and there was no real legal recourse in the event of a dispute.

The third of the revolutions set out by Jones concerns the legal arrangements which were introduced under the Mental Health Act 1959. The new legislation put an end to the lunacy laws and provided for four differing types of patient: the mentally ill, the subnormal, the severely subnormal and those diagnosed as psychopathic. The Act introduced the term 'mental disorder' but it did not define what was meant by mental illness. In short, the Act introduced a number of routes for hospital admission, including admission informally, compulsory admission for observation and separately for treatment. In addition it allowed for admission on the grounds of a psychiatric emergency and for patients already in hospital to be detained for a period against their will. The new legislation also brought in some legal safeguards for patients. In particular, it created the Mental Health Review Tribunal giving patients admitted for treatment a right of appeal against their continued detention. As before, the key professional actors continued to play a leading role as experts in the care of the mentally ill. Medical recommendations were required for compulsory admissions and the social worker was renamed the 'mental welfare officer' for the purposes of the legislation. The Act did not provide for any coherent pattern of service to bring together those involved in the care of an individual patient. It also failed to address the central weakness of the 1946 and 1948 legislation. If the provision of a procedural legal framework constitutes a revolution then the Mental Health Act 1959, was one-third of the three 'revolutions' in mental health social policy of the 1950s. The view taken here is that the case is not only unproven, but to continue to argue for it adds to the myth of the transformation of mental health care in Britian in the 1950s. Such an approach not only contrasted sharply with the daily life experience of thousands of patients in the 1950s and after, but it continues to mock those patients and professionals who live with inadequate and partially developed services today.

## HOSPITALS, PATIENT NUMBERS AND DRUGS

Understanding the changes in policy and practice in the 1950s is important to our grasp of services in the 1990s as much of the thinking of that period forms the roots of current policy and practice. Warner (1985) in his study of recovery from schizophrenia examined 68 follow-up studies of outcomes in Europe and North America. He concluded that recovery rates for patients admitted since the introduction of anti-psychotic drugs are no better than for those admitted after the Second World War or during the first two decades of the century. Warner goes on to argue that there is evidence to show that both the absolute numbers of mental hospital patients and the rates of admission were in decline prior to the drug innovations of the 1950s. This challenges the idea of a 'revolution' in outcomes for patients arising from changes in prescribing.

There are two other arguments which can be made in addition to those put forward by Warner. First, the nineteenth century asylum population and the twentieth century mental hospital populations may be radically different in character. As has been shown earlier the majority of asylum residents were pauper lunatics and their key characteristic was their poverty rather than their mental condition. The asylum became one of a variety of institutions to house them. In the twentieth century with the emergence of psychiatry as a branch of medicine, the ability to diagnose mental illness has become more accurate, codified and consistent; as a result admissions for social reasons have reduced.

The second issue which arises from the Warner study is to question the assumption that the aim of the changes in practice in the 1940s and 1950s was to effect cures. If the aim was improved management of patients in hospital and the community rather than cure then the outcome studies would have to be looked at in a new light. If new techniques and treatments could result in changed patient behaviour then the prospects of improved outcomes within the hospital, such as reduced violence and less seclusion were possible. This was a more modest change than one which would constitute a revolution in practice. It can also be argued that chronically underfunded community care provision had a similar effect in that it reduces the emphasis on the need for a range of services; this in turn can lead to a displacement of people with mental illness into other subgroups of the population such as prison inmates and the homeless and rootless. Warner's study is a serious and coherent review of policy and practice which tries to unmask the underlying political, economic and health issues which inform our understanding of schizophrenia.

## ALL CHANGE? RUNNING DOWN THE OLD HOSPITALS

The expression 'running down' has two distinct meanings in the context of mental health services immediately after the passing of the Mental Health Act 1959. The new legislation created expectations for change at the beginning of the 1960s, particularly with regard to the old hospitals. Many of the ideas and problems being confronted at that time remain unresolved.

The first of the meanings of the term 'running down' was to do with the sense of unease which persisted and increased regarding the purpose of the mental hospitals and the quality of life they afforded for their resident patients. The *Annual*

*Reports of the Ministry of Health* throughout the 1950s and early 1960s record the continued catalogue of problems experienced within the mental hospitals; in particular they note the difficulties of overcrowding and low cost associated with mental hospital care when compared to acute mental specialties. In part this was to do with the much lower 'hotel' costs achieved in the mental hospitals. In many of the institutions they continued to operate as self-sufficient communities with an unpaid labour force growing produce. In spite of this view of mental health services there were a number of innovative and even radical alternative approaches being developed. Examples include the well-documented experiments in Worthing where, after 1955, there was a district mental health service which provided day treatment, psychotherapy and ECT administered in an out-patient setting. The net effect of this approach coupled with an active teaching was a marked reduction in the use of in-patient care for local residents, especially the elderly.

Such work and results as achieved in Worthing, and the new approaches in other areas such as York, Oldham and Birmingham, gave rise to a new sense of therapeutic optimism. It also raised two other key issues. The first was the notion that a mental health service delivered with a community focus was not only desirable, but might actually be more effective. Secondly, these changes called into question the future of the isolated mental hospital as a necessary part of a changing service. Ironically, some of the newly developed approaches to the provision of services actually emphasized the role of institutional life as a force for change. In particular, the rising therapeutic community sought to understand and harness the qualities of institutional life in order to change behaviour. The war-time experience of Dr Maxwell Jones and the work of the Industrial Rehabilitation Units looked to use the persuasive and even coercive characteristics of the institutions to aid patients. One of the key points of these developments was that they made clear that mental health services were not reducible to psychiatry, the medical arm of a range of professions which provided services in hospitals and in the community. In the 1990s it is easy to take for granted the idea that services are provided by teams from a range of disciplines which have an interdependent relationship. Such a view in the 1950s was only partially developed and raised issues of professional rivalry and power in the management of the patient. Some of these issues have proved to be persistent and in the 1990s they form the basis for many relationships in mental health services.

At the heart of the search for alternative approaches to the use of the large old hospital isolated from local communities was a belief that the very 'success' of the institutions was their greatest shortcoming. In a number of books in the late 1950s and early 1960s the institution itself came to be regarded as part of the problem. The 'well-institutionalized' patient was a term used at one time with a sense of approval, whereas by the time of the new legislation in 1959 it was increasingly recognized as a negative consequence of this form of care. The range of critics was considerable and amongst the best known is Barton's (1959) work on institutional neurosis and that of Goffman (1961).

The second meaning attributed to 'running down' the mental hospitals has to do with the scale of operation and in particular the numbers of hospitals and beds they provided. The idea that a 'revolution' had taken place in medical practice through the use of new medication was quickly accepted as a starting point by the Ministry of Health in the planning of new mental health services.

The single most influential piece of work was produced by Tooth and Brooke (1961). This statistical analysis showed that the number of occupied beds had fallen from 3.4 per 1000 in 1954 to 3.1 per 1000 by 1960. Using this approach the figures were then projected forward suggesting that 0.9 beds per 1000 would be needed for patients staying in hospital for less than 2 years. In addition a further 0.9 beds per 1000 population would be needed for the 'new long-stay' patients. This research and the extrapolated figures formed the basis for a new planned approach by central government. In a White Paper entitled a *Hospital Plan for England and Wales* (Ministry of Health, 1962), the Tooth and Brooke figures were transformed into a new statement of intent on the future of the mental hospitals. In the plan it was argued that the need for beds was likely to be 1.8 per 1000 population by 1975 in contrast to 3.4 per 1000 in 1954. The 1960s did see a marked reduction in the total numbers of beds used for mental patients and by 1968 there were 20 000 fewer beds being used for the mentally ill. There are, however, a number of problems with both the basis of the Tooth and Brooke analysis and with the way it was subsequently used by the Ministry of Health. The statistics tell us nothing of the range of needs of patients in the hospital system at the start of the study, in fact the analysis tells us nothing about the people at all other than the bald figures on admissions and discharge rates.

## LIFE AFTER THE ASYLUMS

Given the lessons of the first few years of the NHS and the report of the Royal Commission which preceded the 1959 Act it is surprising that virtually no reference is made to the need for a range of community-based services which work together with hospital services. As to the use made of the research by central government it is questionable if the full implications of the contraction policy of the 1962 plan were considered. Whilst it may be attractive to dispense with institutional provision, at least two significant problems remain. How would those patients who continued to live in the hospital on a long-stay basis be cared for in light of the new therapeutic optimism? Of those 110 000 patients identified in the original 1954 group some 30 000 were still in hospital almost two decades later. Of this residual group almost half were elderly. For them the statistical projections and the new hospital planning system did little or nothing.

Part of the three 'revolutions' referred to earlier was the development of so-called 'open door' policies to facilitate access to services in the mental hospital. As part of the emerging therapeutic optimism of the 1950s which was associated with the new drug technology there was a shift towards the earlier discharge of psychotic patients. Conditions which previously necessarily involved long, open-ended periods of in-patient care were treated more rapidly. Perhaps it would be more accurate to say that there was a marked increase in medical confidence to manage the symptoms of such conditions. This lead to renewed emphasis on the importance of early diagnosis and assessment and a belief in the efficiency of rehabilitation for people with mental illness.

The belief in earlier intervention coupled with a concerted policy of after-care and rehabilitation lead to two important developments. The first was an increased use of a range of other disciplines and professions in mental health care; these included Occupational Therapy and Psychology both of which took leading roles in the creation of rehabilitative approaches to mental illness. The second of these changes, the emergence of 'open door' policies was more complex. In contrast to traditional mental health policies and the stigma associated with mental hospital admission the new-found aim of public policy was to facilitate easier access to services. This in turn lead to a change in the way hospitals were used as the task was increasingly seen as admission for treatment and discharge rather than containment and incarceration. This led rapidly to the emergence of the 'revolving door' practice which was to become a consistent feature of mental hospitals after the 1950s. It meant that the total numbers of hospital patients was reduced but the new population is made up of a significant number of people who pass through the system time and time again. This in turn posed problems for the management of patients whose illness was episodic in character, especially where the principal device available to professionals was the in-patient service of the hospital set apart from continuing services in the community.

## COMMUNITY CARE: THE MYTHICAL ALTERNATIVE

It has become increasingly common to polarize the institution and the community as two absolute and alternative means of providing mental health services. The cases are often parodies of the complexity of the real world of individual patient needs and care. However such simple distinctions serve as powerful weapons in attacking or defending particular approaches to service. The type of simple polemic used to justify or criticize hospital or community provision is set out in Table 3.1.

**Table 3.1** Characteristics of community and institutional care

| Type of care | Characteristics | |
| | Positive | Negative |
| --- | --- | --- |
| Asylum | A refuge providing protection | Coercive and stigmatizing |
| Community | Caring and enabling neighbourhood | Uncaring and exploitative |

In this view the institutional care provided by the hospital can be justified as a place of safety and respite from a hostile outside world of a community which only exists as a desire not a reality. To those who take the community position the use of institutional care can be de-skilling and an isolating experience which not only adds little to the patient's life-chance but also positively works against him when it is time to leave the institution. There is a third strand to this argument which is shared by both sides of this debate and that is to do with the costs and benefits of each approach. Both the hospital-based model of care and the community approach look to the resources tied up in the opposing services and make claims about the quality of work which could be achieved if the monies were not used for other services but invested in their preferred approach. Much of this debate is conducted in a sterile and unproductive atmosphere which ensures that the issues of coordinated care for patients and clients figure little in the discussion. Such posturing and caricaturing of others' approaches is most damaging when it occurs between differing agencies who need to be working together towards common aims. In such circumstances it is only the patient or the client who ultimately suffers. It is these views and those like them which powerfully influence the day-to-day experience of users of the mental health system. In both the hospital/institution and the community alternative, it may well be that the actual experience is different from the external appearance and this may result in the best quality work being conducted in the most unpromising circumstances.

One of the alternatives to the old style asylum which had developed by the early 1960s was the appearance of Departments of Psychiatry within local District General Hospitals. One of the arguments in their favour was that it would serve to integrate mental illness services with other parts of the NHS. Whilst it is undoubtedly true it is a partial response to a much more complex problem which involved future of provisions for the long-stay patient, the development of alternative strategies to hospital admission and the coordination of services with agencies based outside the hospital.

## TAKING THE PLACE OF THE ASYLUMS

Before proceeding further with an account of the emergence of official community care policies it is worth considering what care in the community sought to replace. The old hospitals were not a comprehensive mental health service as they provided only for those who were admitted to the institutions. Consequently there was no other form of provision available and if there was a need for care, the patient was admitted. Chapter 1 set out some of the problems created for those who were admitted; not least among them was the dual difficulty of legal certification and subsequent social stigma. However it is important to understand what the large old hospitals did provide and to look at how the positive features of the institutions could be reproduced in community-based services. The asylums did provide shelter, food, companionship and recreation, albeit on a scale and in a form that few people would freely choose to receive. In short, the asylums provided the necessities of life often at a price which many regard as unacceptably high. That price was the loss of focus on the individual patient and their unique and special needs. If the new approach of the 1960s was to succeed it would have to provide the positive features of the old hospitals as well as the attractions of a well-resourced community system which integrated health and social provision for each individual patient. For many people who work in or receive mental health services today, the idea of a comprehensive and integrated service remains an aspiration.

In light of these comments it is possible to reformulate Table 3.1 to take into account the development of mental health services in hospital settings; separate from the function of asylum. The crude contrast of local communities as either caring or indifferent is not an accurate depiction of the complexity of the real world. The model set out in Table 3.1 needs to be recast to take account of the range of services and functions which have developed since the 1950s as well as the emergence of changing perceptions of health and social care for people with mental illness (Table 3.2). It is important that none of the approaches is set out in such a way that they are a parody of themselves, but clearly representatives of this type are convenient, shorthand attempts to capture and compare services.

The discussion so far has been about the demise of the approach to the provision for the mentally ill which was inherited from the Victorians. Special attention has been given to the changing perception and role of the large old hospitals

**Table 3.2** Characteristics of institutional and community provision

| | Characteristics | |
| Type of care | Positive | Negative |
| --- | --- | --- |
| Asylum/institution provision | Refuge, shelter and protection | Coercive and stigmatizing |
| District hospital services | Manages symptoms | Drug-centred |
| Community care services | Caring and enabling | Uncaring and exploitative |

as the single vehicle for the provision of mental health services. Dr John Wing commented in an article on the functions of asylum in the *British Journal of Psychiatry* (1990) that scandals which now feature in the press occur in the 'community' rather than in the hospitals. Wing contrasts the function of asylum as a process with the old asylum buildings which are part of the structure of mental health services. He asks whether the function of asylum can be provided without an asylum as one component of a district service?

THE DRIFT TOWARDS CARE IN THE COMMUNITY

If the notion of community care has proved to be difficult to both describe and achieve, why has it been discussed and pursued with such intensity for over four decades? Despite this activity it has still to be achieved to the satisfaction of any of the parties in the debate. One way of beginning to explore this quesiton is to look at some of the issues and forces which encouraged the search for an alternative to the old hospital system. The answer to this seemingly simple question is rich and complex even if the explanation leaves aside the issue of motivation. There are five identifiable factors:

1. **Economics.** The old hospitals were only viable within their allocated budgets if they could be run on low unit cost per patient. This could be partly achieved by the use of an unpaid labour-force from within the patient population. As alternative approaches began to develop and the pattern of hospital admissions changed, it became evident that the

hospitals were increasingly likely to be dealing with a more dependent and ageing population who were unable to labour. With such a patient group the cost of nursing and support service was likely to increase to a point where the unit costs were unacceptable for the standard of care provided.

2. **Changing perceptions.** Much had been achieved in trying to undo the stigma associated with mental illness. Campaigns ran throughout the 1950s to reduce the fears and misconceptions associated with the nineteenth century view of insanity. Legal changes had facilitated easier access to mental health services, both procedurally and organizationally, in such a way that by the 1950s and 1960s increasing numbers of patients were admitted informally for short periods. In addition, new methods of treatment such as psychotherapy were perceived as less authoritarian and invasive than detention or drug therapies. However, some of the old problem of stigma proved to be persistent despite changes in the way the hospitals were used and the range of new services which were developing.

3. **New services.** Increasingly, the work which was being applauded as innovative and fresh was taking place outside the isolated institutions and as a consequence there was a growing tendency to regard the asylums as backwaters which were no more than warehouses for long-stay patients.

4. **Professional power.** Most of the profesional groups in mental health services had organized themselves sufficiently after the war to develop a coherent view on social policy, as witnesssed by the volume and quality of the evidence submitted to the Royal Commission which preceded the 1959 Act. No longer were the doctors, nurses and psychiatric social workers to remain rooted in the institutions separate from the public debates taking place in wider society. For the doctors and nurses, particularly, this development must have been something of a double-edged sword, as they had successfully professionalized themselves as experts in the care of the mentally ill *within* the asylums. It was this very institutional base, which had served them for over a century, which was increasingly seen as an obstacle to greater acceptance in the rest of the NHS.

5. **The isolation of the asylums.** The last of the factors is perhaps the most uncomfortable and the most fickle. Public opinion on mental health services had for years been shaped by the asylums and the use of detention with its implicit associations with custody and danger. What had not stopped over the years was the catalogue of scandals and malpractice associated with institutional care. Even though such reports were statistically infrequent they fuelled public anxieties and perceptions which vacillated between wildly contrasting stereotypes of easy cures or hopeless incarceration.

### CHANGE FROM ABOVE: GOVERNMENT INITIATIVES

Fifteen years after the new Hospital Plan which had followed hard on the heels of the new mental health legislation there was a major government review of mental health policy and practice. The Ministry of Health had been superceded by a new government Department of Health and Social Security. This body which brought together the three strands of health, social services and social security into a single department was characteristic of central government of the period which made a feature of central planning and control by amalgamating differing government functions under new umbrella organizations. The result of this review was *Better Services for the Mentally Ill* which was presented to parliament in 1975 (Department of Health, 1975). The foreword by Barbara Castle, Secretary of State for Social Services opened by referring to mental illness as 'perhaps the major health problem of our time' (p. ii) and it then goes on to discuss the impact of mental illness on the economy through lost days at work. The politician's comments make reference to the problems associated with the funding of the community care approach, especially the need to set clear policy objectives against which priorities could be assessed.

The opening comments of the white paper now appear to be prophetic as it is clearly stated that the status of the proposals is that of a long-term strategic plan. Mrs Castle was emphatic that the paper was not a specific programme for implementation but rather a broad statement of the general direction for social policy. This approach set out clearly the fact that local services would have to continue for some years to be based on existing mental hospitals. Reading these comments again almost two decades later the position has changed only marginally in that the two thrusts for change, the integration of health and social services and the development of community-based services still remain out of reach for patients and practitioners alike.

*Better Services for the Mentally Ill* argued that the general approach of community care remained valid and the future aims of services should continue to emphasize the development of much more locally-based services, as well as a shift in the balance from hospital to social services-based care. Psychiatric services were encouraged to develop in the district general hospitals but there was a warning note sounded about the risk of creaming off those patients who were likely to make quicker progress and in turn create a two-tier system with the old mental hospitals as isolated institutions. It is difficult to see why this was feared as a possibility when it was already becoming a reality. The paper is careful not to eulogize community care unquestioningly as it warns against assuming that 'communities' are simply geographical. The uncertainty commented on in the document regarding the future of the mental hospitals originated in official thinking in the 1962 Hospital Plan. However the review carefully distinguishes between three alternative futures for the mental hospitals. Some were said to be capable of being phased out quickly, others would have a reduced role and a proportion would have a continuing major role in the long term. What the report does not say is on what criteria these distinctions would be made or what were the funding implications. For those hospitals which were likely to continue in use there was no talk of the necessary investment programme to give the buildings a life in the long term nor was there any discussion of the investment in staff development which would be required. The uncertainty in the funding and resources for the mentally ill also highlighted a schism in official thinking as regards priority groups in need of services. The 1970s saw an unprecedented expansion in the role of the new local authority social services department. However the investments were not made in services for the mentally ill but rather in child care services and in residential provision for the elderly. The level of funding by the local authorities will be discussed in a later chapter when considering the current problems of planning and integrating services between agencies.

The review of mental health services was prospective in the approach it took to the future of service, especially in the need for coordinated services and the respective roles of health and social services. The report sought to expand social services' provision in residential care, day care and social work support. In addition it looked to move specialist services into more accessible local settings and create organizational links between social services and health staff in terms of primary care and planning. In 1975 the term 'manager' was virtually unknown in the language of the caring professions in either health or social services.

The paper proposed another change in practice: improvement in staffing levels to enable individual patient care to be assessed on a multi-disciplinary basis, so allowing early intervention and preventative work. To a new entrant to social services or the NHS in the 1990s these ideas and proposals would appear fresh and innovative rather than remnants of a report two decades old. The principal reason for their appeal would not be because of the novel quality of the ideas but because the ambitions of 1975 have yet to be realized. For those people who received services in the expanding residential care sector of the local authority, the reality today is unlikely to be optimistic. The accrual of a significant proportion of elderly dementing residents being cared for by poorly trained auxiliary staff is a far cry from the multi-disciplinary promise of 1975.

The White Paper was a curious mixture of an insightful commentary on the changes in attitude and provision over a 15-year period and a cynical recognition of the political and economic obstacles to further change. An example of this can be found in the section on the role of the social services. The White Paper comments that:

> The development of residential, day care, and social work support services must be co-ordinated. From the patient's point of view, discharge from hospital to a community which lacks the hospital's facilities for day-time shelter and occupation may well be a change for the worse.
>
> *(para 4.22, p. 34)*

In less than 50 words the report described the world which was to face practitioner and patient alike throughout the

1970s, 1980s and on into the 1990s. The same simple sentences served as a good precis of the key political agenda for social policy for the 1990s with the emphasis on working together, coordination and planning.

With such an emphasis on the role of services based in the community, including psychiatric services in the general hospital; what did the White Paper have to say about those patients who were thought to need long-term care? The report distinguished between two groups of patient the 'old' long-stay and the 'new' long-stay. Of the 104 000 patients in mental hospitals identified in the 1971 census some 75 000 had been in hospital for more than one year. Of this group more than half (57%) had been in hospital for more than 10 years and of these over one-third (39%) had been in hospital for more than 20 years. It was recognized by the report that many of these patients remained in hospital for two principal reasons. First, they had become fully institutionalized and it would be both difficult and unjust to try to move such people on. Second, the means and resources to resettle this group of patients simply did not exist and was unlikely to exist in the foreseeable future. The Paper acknowledged frankly that given the same presenting problems by the 1980s the use of long-stay hospital care was seen as inappropriate for many of these patients. The White Paper also commented on the 'new' long-stay patients. In 1971 there were just over 21 000 patients who had been in mental hospitals for 1–5 years and this did not include elderly patients suffering from dementia. Out of this report and subsequent research studies arose the development of the hospital hostel ward which provided 24-hour nursing cover, in smaller units than the acute wards. These became a feature of health service thinking in the late 1970s and early 1980s as an alternative to using back wards in the old mental hospitals, and to free beds in the acute sector.

### THE MENTAL HEALTH ACT 1983:
### MISSED OPPORTUNITIES FOR CHANGE

The central government Hospital Plan of 1962 appeared shortly after the introduction of the Mental Health Act 1959, and the 1975 White Paper was produced as an overall reassessment of the services for the mentally ill. The publication of an official review of mental health policy stimulated a new climate of change. Expectations were raised for those who worked in the mental hospitals, departments of psychiatry and in community services to expect significant changes in both the pace and direction of mental health policy. What actually resulted was the Mental Health Act 1983, which did little to address the fundamental issues of fragmented services and chronic under-funding which has festered since 1948. The promise of the 1975 review lead to a sense of anticlimax in that the focus of change was once again to concentrate on the legal conditions which informed mental health provision. What was needed in the view of those working in the field was a thorough reform of the structure and process of mental health provision. The challenge had been thrown down by the 1975 review, albeit couched in cautious parliamentary language. The response to the review (the 1983 Act) missed both the point of the problem and the opportunities open at the time. Before looking at the problems set up by this renewed attention to the legal framework rather than to services it is worth reiterating the main features of the 1983 Act as it informs important parts of current practice, especially for a minority of patients who require compulsory in-patient treatment. Table 3.3 shows the six main routes for compulsory hospital admission under the Part II of the Mental Health Act 1983.

Whilst the 1983 Act does not define mental illness it uses a broad category of mental disorder throughout the legislation. The use of compulsory detention is set out in Part II of the Act and as well as providing detailed requirements for the use of admission procedures, the Act also sets out the arrangements for discharge of patients (s. 23). Patients who have been compulsorily admitted can be discharged through actions instigated by the hospital managers, the nearest relatives, the Mental Health Review Tribunal (Section 72) or after a specific period of time has elapsed (ss. 18 and 17). Hospital managers may prevent an application by a nearest relative after taking medical advice from the responsible medical officer in charge of the patient's care.

Two of the most controversial forms of treatment appear in Part IV of the Mental Health Act and these are psycho-surgery which was widely practised in Britain and America in the 1930s, but has now become relatively rare; and surgical

**Table 3.3** Compulsory admission criteria

| Section | Purpose | Duration | Grounds | Procedure |
|---|---|---|---|---|
| 2 | Assessment | Up to 28 days | Patient suffers from a mental disorder which in the interest of his own health and safety or with a view to the protection of other persons, warrants his detention in hospital for assessment for at least a limited period | Application by nearest relative or approved social worker. Requires two medical recommendations, one of whom is approved |
| 3 | Treatment | Initially for 6 months but can be extended for 1-year periods | Patient suffers from mental illness, severe mental impairment, psychopathic disorder or mental impairment that makes it appropriate for him to receive treatment in hospital and: (i) in the case of psychopathic disorder or mental impairment, such treatment is likely to alleviate or prevent further deterioration of his condition; and (ii) it is necessary for the health or safety of the patient or for the protection of other persons that he should receive such treatment, and it cannot be provided unless he is detained under this section | As section 2 above |
| 4 | Emergency assessment | Up to 72 hours | Admission for assessment is urgently necessary and compliance with section 2 would cause undesirable delay | Application by nearest relative or approved social worker. Requires one medical recommendation |

**Table 3.3** *cont'd*

| Section | Purpose | Duration | Grounds | Procedure |
|---|---|---|---|---|
| 5(2) | To detain an informal patient already in hospital | Up to 72 hours | In the view of the doctor in charge of the the patient's treatment, informal status is no longer appropriate | The medical practitioner currently responsible for the patient |
| 5(4) | Nurse's holding power | Up to 6 hours | Patient is suffering from a mental disorder to such a degree that it is necessary for his health or safety, or for the protection of others, for him to be immediately restrained from leaving hospital. It is not practicable to secure the immediate attendance of a practitioner for the purpose of furnishing a report under section 5(2) | Application by a Registered Mental Nurse |
| 7 | Guardian-ship | As section 3 above | Application is necessary in the interest of the welfare of the patient that he should be received into the guardianship of the local social services department | Application by nearest relative or by the approved social worker. Requires two medical recommen-dations, one of whom is approved |

implantation of hormones to reduce the male sex drive in cases of mental disorder. Both of these forms of treatment require that involvement of a medical officer appointed by the Secretary of State under section 57 of the Act. The section and subsequent treatment is required to meet three conditions: the patient's consent, clarification that the patient is capable of consenting and a certificate to show that the treatment is likely to be beneficial. If the patient refuses consent, is incapable of consent or there is uncertainty about the benefits of the treatment then consent is withheld. The responsible medical officer must inform the Mental Health Act Commissioners of the intention to offer this treatment and an independent second medical opinion is appointed by the Secretary of State. In addition, two other persons who are not doctors are also appointed to ensure that if consent is given it is valid within the meaning of the Act.

For detained patients who are said to require the continued use of a medicine or ECT then the Act provides for this (s. 58). Unlike section 57, the consent to treatment rules of section 58 allows for the doctor to over-rule the patient given that second opinion has been sought from two people professionally concerned with the patient's treatment. One of these people must be a nurse.

The question of consent to treatment raises a number of legal and moral questions which are not easily resolved. How can it be shown that the unprotesting and compliant patient is freely giving consent to treatment. Equally, if the patient freely gives consent for ECT then how should clinical staff respond part way through the procedure if the patient protests his/her refusal? Such circumstnaces are legally and professionally worrying for all concerned, especially when it is essential to continue a trusting relationship with a patient over a long period.

One of the remnants from the eighteenth century vagrancy laws relates to mentally disordered persons found in a public place. Under the terms of the Act (s. 136) a police constable has the power to remove the person to a place of safety such as a hospital or a police station. Perhaps the most curious section of the Act is that which relates to those patients not admitted on a compulsory basis, i.e. the majority of all patients receiving mental hospital care. The Act provides for easy access on an informal admission basis at the patient's request (s. 131) but sets this out almost as an afterthought rather than as the principal route into hospital care for the majority of patients admitted. What is even more surprising is that the Act does not even acknowledge the role of all other forms of intervention such as out-patients and day care or the services of new forms of community support.

There are two other provisions in the Mental Health Act which are significant for those who work and live within the current arrangements and as points of principal. Reference has already been made to the Mental Health Act Commissioners and Mental Health Review Tribunals. The Commissioners essentially are the link to the Board of Control and the Commissioners on Lunacy before them. They act as an inspectorate for the mental health system but only in respect of detained patients. The role of the Commissioners is essentially limited to annual inspection and as such they are unable to develop a more sustained relationship with any particular service. This limitation has been accentuated because administratively, they are now a centralized service whereas they used to operate from regional centres. Mental Health Review Tribunals act as a source of appeal for patients detained under the terms of the Act and as such they suffer from the same problem as the commissioners. They focus their attention on a subject of the small minority of patients cared for in hospitals – those compulsorily detained under the Mental Health Act.

BUSINESS AS USUAL: THE LIMITS OF THE 1983 ACT

The question which needs to be addressed is to what degree did the Act of 1983 help to resolve the new problems faced by mental health professionals and service-users? In a number of vital respects the 1983 Act is similar to the 1959 Act. The legal framework for mental health policy has not kept pace with thinking within practice, neither has it recognized the contribution of patients' and relatives' organizations in improving mental health care. The perspective which dominated thinking in the drafting of the legislation was that of the hospital as an institution and the need to compulsorily detain people with mental illness in hospital. The approved social worker has the role of functionary in the Act and is caught between having some specialist knowledge of the mentally ill and the legal role of making applications for hospital admission. It is questionable whether the mentally ill receive a better social work service from the 'approved social worker' of the 1980s onwards than they did from the old 'mental welfare officer' of the 1960s. The Act simply does not provide the means to develop standards of good practice, especially in the area of preventative work.

Mental health services are depicted in the 1983 Act as narrow legal procedures which proscribe professional behaviour narrowly. Just as this approach can be argued to be an effective deterrent against bad practice, so it fails to encourage innovative or good practice. In the narrow view of the legislation the world of mental health services concentrate on hospital care and the loss of liberty. There is little or no account taken of work of new forms of care in acute services, psychiatry of old age or for people with enduring mental illness. The place of the doctor continues, as before the 1959 Act and the 1983 legislation, as the expert in mental health problems. The Act itself does nothing to encourage good mental health practice which allows the doctor to work jointly with other disciplines, the non-statutory sector, the patient and relatives to manage care and minimize the degree of disruption brought on by illness. *The Code of Practice* (Department of Health and Welsh Office, 1990) which followed some 6 years after the Act itself attempts to redress this balance by providing examples of good practice and developing a fuller set of explanations of the ways in which the act can be interpreted. The most regrettable part of the law is that it does not reflect either the day-to-day experience of patients, in that it does not protect their rights, nor does it recognize that most people agree to receiving mental health care.

The Mental Health Act 1983 was a case of a missed opportunity to put right problems which had been identified decades before. Services for the mentally ill were fragmented between local authority provision and the NHS; there was neither the structure nor the process to ensure that the complex needs of individual patients or clients were jointly discussed, let alone met. Chapter 4 will look at attempts to address the issues in mental health and welfare policies and practices which the changes of 1983 failed to consider.

# 4

# Radical conservatism

## HEALTH, SOCIAL CARE AND THE NEW POLITICS

The period from 1979 to 1990 in British politics was dominated by the values, attitudes and personality of Margaret Thatcher whose personal views became the new orthodoxy of the Conservative Party. 'Thatcherism' radically challenged the Conservative Party's policies and beliefs formed after 1945.

Before Thatcherism, the Conservative Party had been dominated by a set of beliefs which arose from their defeat in the 1945 general election. Their social and economic policies after the war were designed to win the peace, electorally. These ideas on health, education, housing and industrial development are now conveniently grouped together as 'one-nation' conservatism. What is usually meant by this term in the context of health care policy is an acceptance of the idea of a mixed economy of public and private provision within the National Health Service. The dominant assumption was that there was a legitimate role for the state as a key provider of health and welfare services, free at the point of delivery. This policy also allowed for the provision of private health care and education should it be preferred by those who could afford it. The emphasis was on the place of individual choice rather than the single option of the state service freely available to all. The 'one-nation' conservatives were led by the young Turks of the Party, including Iain MacLeod and Enoch Powell, both of whom were Ministers of Health in the 1950s and 1960s.

Underpinning the approach of post-war conservatism was an attempt to set aside class conflict and bring to an end the idea that political parties represented particular class interests.

The Conservative Party set out to produce policies which had the look of universal appeal to people from all social classes, in contrast to the Labour Party which saw the problem of reconstruction in terms of increasing the role of the state in economic activity and domestic social policy 'to reduce class inequalities'. The Conservatives emphasized an end to class distinction rather than narrowing the gap between classes. Throughout the 1950s the process of economic recovery continued superficially as never before. Individual wealth for the majority of people expanded as never before. The government oversaw record numbers of public sector houses being built along with an expansion in the number of universities and places of higher education. Under this veneer of affluence, however, the British economy was in serious decline. The ability of the British economy to grow in a sustained way without the cycle of boom and recession had not been achieved. Personal wealth for many had been achieved in the short term without a corresponding investment in the renewal of the industrial base of the country. Despite winning the military war, Britain was slowly but steadily losing the peace. British industry was increasingly uncompetitive and consistently failed over the following three decades to invest in the industrial base. Many industries fell into decline and eventually either lost their identity or folded completely. One of the casualties of this process was the Conservative Party itself, which despite the belief in the attractions of the 'one-nation' approach, proved unable to manage the ailing economy of the late 1950s.

By the early 1960s there was a sense that the Conservative Party was out of touch with both the needs of the country and the views of the voters. The result was that the Conservative Party lost parliamentary power for most of the 1960s to the Labour Party led by Harold Wilson. The Labour Party emphasized the potential of the new technology as the means to revitalize British industry to achieve better living standards and social stability. Whilst these ideas and beliefs may well have been well-founded, the reality was in sharp contrast.

Despite winning two general elections in the 1960s the Labour Party became increasingly embroiled in economic crisis which resulted in a sterling crisis and a devaluation of the pound and increased public borrowing. The Conservatives won power again in 1970 under the leadership of Edward

Heath who shared the 'one-nation' view, but who also held
strong beliefs on the need for Britain to be an equal partner
in the expanding European Economic Community. The Heath
government witnessed a period of major industrial conflict with
workers in the public sector and the nationalized industries
involved in widespread strikes and drawn-out pay claims. In
1974 there were two general elections which resulted in the Conservatives winning in February 1974 and losing power to the
Labour Party in October 1974. Both political parties subsequently
changed leaders with Wilson giving way to Jim Callaghan and
Heath to Margaret Thatcher. From 1974 to 1979 the Labour Party
was in office with the Conservatives in opposition; both parties,
however, were faced with the same two questions: what policies
would bring continued electoral victory and what could be done
to arrest declining industrial performance?

The years from the mid to the late 1970s were some of the
unhappiest for the Labour Party, despite the fact that they held
office. The Party was continually beset with internal
disagreements as well as economic pressures to restrict and
reduce public expenditure, including health and welfare
programmes. Paradoxically it was in the low-paid sections of
the public sector where industrial unrest was most active. The
most publicized results of these competing pressures was the
1979 'winter of discontent' which saw significant industrial relations' problems emerge in the public sector. Callaghan chose
to call a general election as a vote of confidence in the Labour
government. Labour lost the election and this heralded a new
style of radical Conservatism under the leadership of Margaret
Thatcher. The Thatcher years in office from 1979 to 1990 had two
qualities which were absent from the Labour and Conservative
administrations of the 1970s; Thatcher's governments proved
to be radical policy-makers and comprehensive in their approach
to government. To understand both the form and content of
changes in the health service, especially in the late 1980s requires
an understanding of what is meant by 'Thatcherism' and the
impact it made on all aspects of life in Britain.


ECONOMIC PERFORMANCE: SOCIAL WELFARE AND GOVERNMENT

It has already been argued that, in the nineteenth century,
mental health policy was one of a number of social issues which

served as a battle ground for competing views on the proper role of government. The key questions in these debates focused on two central issues. The first concerned the degree to which the state should intervene in society as a whole? The second was to establish the relationship between the rights of the individual and the power of the state. For 35 years after the Second World War British governments had been elected to oversee a mixed economy of health care within the context of the Welfare State. The role of government was to ensure that basic services were provided along with a safety net for those who needed protection or were unable to care for themselves. Broadly speaking, the approach to health and welfare was the same as support to industry. In manufacturing, basic services were provided through the use of nationalized industries or by the use of subsidies. By the time the first Thatcher government came to power in 1979 economic decline was well under way in Britain. The previous strategies of Conservative and Labour governments had failed to stop the cycle of economic boom and bust which had characterized British post-war economic performance.

In 1979 there was no well-articulated doctrine called 'Thatcherism' which could be examined and criticized. What emerged over the first 3 years of the administration was an approach which emphasized personal effort and entrepreneurial ability, a shift from state provision to the private sector and a move from traditional manufacturing to the service industries such as financial services. There was a parallel and complimentary approach being developed in America by the Reagan administration which not only emphasized the individual and personal responsibility, but also cut welfare programmes. Like Thatcher, Reagan took the view that social problems were not a result of social inequality or social deprivation but rather a form of deviance which resulted from poor personal performance. Thatcher followed the logic of her own argument and even questioned the existance of society itself. The style of government and social policy was very personal to Margaret Thatcher and as a result there was little room for dissent within the Thatcher cabinet. By the end of the Thatcher years not one single minister who served in the 1979 cabinet remained in office, other than the Prime Minister herself.

The deep-seated economic depression of the late 1970s continued for the early part of Thatcher's first administration, although electorally the party was successful. In 1982 Britain became involved in an undeclared war with Argentina over claims to the Falkland Islands in the South Atlantic. As a result of the military victory and a growing sense of national confidence the Conservative Party won another general election. The platform for this victory was the emerging doctrine of 'Thatcherism' which was beginning to make a real impact on social policy as well as industry. One of the core themes of the new Tory radicalism was a dread of individuals becoming dependent on the state. This belief led directly to major reforms of the social security system which switched many benefits from automatic status to discretionary decisions of local officers. The Social Fund was created which allowed clients to take out loans which had to be repaid rather than grants which were given. In the housing field one of the most popular policies introduced by the administration was the selling of council houses to residents at discounted prices. The 1950s idea of a property-owning democracy was becoming a reality under a radical Conservative government rather than a Labour government which had long promised change in housing policy. The government introduced a range of measures to 'privatize' industries previously tied to the state. These included basic heavy industries, manufacturing which received government subsidies, public utilities and new technology companies which previously relied on a government stake.

Throughout the 1980s Britain increasingly was run on the lines of an industrial holding company rather than as the traditional mixed economy which had developed over the preceding 40 years. In such a new society there was a much greater emphasis given to the provision of financial services rather than to subsidizing old industries which required major investment. The approach was essentially the *laissez faire* attitude of 'let the market decide'. If people wanted a particular product or service then they should use their buying power to choose it. Conversely, if there is no demand then the company either changes its product or goes out of business. Such a system was fuelled by marked reductions in personal taxation and a consequent reduction in monies available for public expenditure. In addition, there was a significant growth in the use of credit with the underlying risk of rising inflation just below the surface.

Throughout the 1980s unemployment fell, according to the official figures of the Department of Employment, but this masked wholesale changes in the way people earned their living. Many hundreds of thousands of self-employed jobs were created, but many businesses failed. Many of the new jobs were in service industries where much of the work was part time and relatively poorly paid. Substantial reductions were achieved in the numbers of people officially classified as unemployed simply by changing the criteria. Young people on one of the training schemes did not count in the unemployment figures, despite their not having a permanent job. The 1980s also saw the re-emergence of an underclass of people who did not benefit from the new prosperity. Many of these people lived in the inner cities which had suffered either through the 'gentrification' of old residential areas or the shift from town centre retailing to the out-of-town shopping developments. Property development became both a symbol of the new radical politics and the means for many to prosper. Changes in the benefits system, the reduction of subsidized housing for rent, the rising values of old property and the introduction of the 'poll tax' all led to the creation of a disaffected underclass of people in the inner cities who were swept aside by the new pursuit of personal wealth. The results were mixed, ranging from occasional riots in Liverpool, Manchester and Bristol over the living conditions of black Britons in the inner cities, to public disorder in London in protests over the poll tax.

Within this context of fundamental political and economic change was born the idea that it was time to review the state provision of health and welfare services and to initiate a reform programme. This idea, like much of the political and social policy agenda of the 1980s, was the personal view of the Prime Minister. The changes which ensued were to have far-reaching effects on patients, clients, professionals and politicians alike. It is these ideas and changes which will be examined in the next section of this chapter.

## THE WHITE PAPER CHASE: TOWARDS MANAGED CARE

The changes introduced by the Thatcher governments throughout the 1980s were radical in both scale and content and they consisted of two major strands. The first of these was an emphasis on changing people's attitudes and values from a state-managed society to a market-driven society. The second emphasized an action programme to implement the overall goals set out by government. This point highlights one of the real anomalies of radical Conservatism of the period: the government which claimed to reduce the role of the state actually centralized power to a far greater extent than had previously been experienced.

Before going on to explore the two most significant proposals for change, the White Papers on the organization and function of the NHS and the implementation of 'care in the community' policies, it is worth recapping on the steps in the White Paper chase from the middle of the 1970s to the beginning of the 1990s. In all, central government took 12 measures to set the political and professional agenda for health and social care:

1975 *Better Services for the Mentally Ill*
1983 Mental Health Act
1983 *Management Enquiry Report* (Griffiths 1)
1986 Disabled Persons Act
1986 *Making a Reality of Community Care*
1987 *Promoting Better Health*
1988 *Agenda for Action* (Griffiths 2)
1989 *Working for Patients*
1989 *Caring for People*
1990 Code of Practice (Mental Health Act)
1991 Community Care Act
1991 *The Nation's Health*

The reform programme of the Conservative governments of the 1980s developed an identifiable house style which characteristically set out the aims of policy but said little about the means to achieve it. Social policy changed from an administrative process dominated by procedure to a political process driven by clearly-stated ends. The means to achieve these ends were often worked out along the way by those who had to practice within the system. What did become clear were the values and the vision which informed those ends. It was a vision of a market process, where products are made available to consumers and the more business-like survive and prosper. The question facing the Thatcher government, however, and more particularly Margaret Thatcher herself, was how could the new-found enterprise culture be applied to health and welfare services? The problem was particularly difficult given the special status of the NHS in British political life over the last four decades and the political minefield associated with attacks on the Welfare State. The answers to these questions were to set in train a range of reforms which would take the rest of the century to complete whilst still continuing to deliver services to patients and clients.

## THE LANGUAGE OF THE MARKET PLACE

The first move by the Thatcher government to initiate change in the health service was characteristic of the approach adopted in successive years. The Prime Minister appointed Sir Roy Griffiths, the Managing Director of Sainsbury's supermarkets, to examine the way in which the health service was managed and to make recommendations for change. The message was clear for all to hear; the NHS was going to become more business-like and the architect was to be one of Britain's most successful businessmen. Sir Roy Griffiths' report was published in 1983 as the *NHS Management Enquiry Report* and it set out to radically change the way health services were managed. Central to these changes was a series of criticisms of the consensus style of management which the NHS had adopted. Griffiths was especially critical of the way in which multi-disciplinary management teams had failed to provide either strategic or operational leadership to health professionals in planning and service delivery. Griffiths prescription for the NHS was twofold: first establish general management at regional, district and unit levels of the organization and, second, involve medical staff in management. Griffiths was, in effect, looking to introduce a series of measures to change the status of managers from administrators to managers who controlled all aspects of the organization. This meant that, in the new proposals, leadership and control became the personal task of the new general managers whether they had regional, district or unit responsibilities. Part of the Griffiths' message was that managing change was not only the role of management, but it was a natural part of any dynamic organization.

These changes were accepted by the Secretary of State and this first Griffiths Report became the blueprint for the initial wave of change in the health service. For individual managers the changes were profound. They included not only new responsibilities which were subject to a formal annual appraisal system, but also the introduction of 3-year rolling contracts for unit general managers and above, as well as performance-related payments. The Griffiths changes, however, dealt only with the structural and organizational issues in the NHS; they did not deal with the process of managing health care or the relationship between health provision and social care which was available outside the NHS. Equally, the criticism of the 1970s style of consensus management was an implicit attack on the idea of multi-disciplinary working. This was especially evident given the separate role identified by Griffiths for doctors in management. In the mental health field, other professions such as nurses, occupational therapists and social workers had been establishing working relationships based on the multi-disciplinary approach, as a blueprint for better future practice.

With hindsight the 1983 Griffiths Report can be seen as a perceptive and successful attempt to break the mould of traditional health service administration which had failed to plan effectively or control the business side of the organization. Griffiths devolved to managers the power to develop local strategies to enable the health service to adapt to changing circumstances. It can also be said that the Report tended to treat the NHS as if it was all run on the lines of acute hospital-based services. The work of Sir Roy Griffiths in 1983 was only the opening shot in a series of changes in the management and organization of the NHS which developed throughout the 1980s. The impact of these changes are still emerging and they will shape the NHS well into the next century. Amongst the most complicated services to undergo change was the provision for the mentally ill as they involved agencies outside the NHS, as well as those professionals within health who continued to struggle with the nineteenth century legacy described in Chapter 1.

## CHANGING PUBLIC SECTOR PERFORMANCE

The need for change in both the pace and direction of services was recognized by the Audit Commission (1986) in *Making a Reality of Community Care* which reviewed progress on provision in the community since the 1975 White Paper referred to earlier. The Audit Commissioners' report produced evidence to show that less than one-third of the planned day centres and less than half the required day hospitals had been created. The report was critical of the relationships between the health authorities and the social services' departments, especially in planning matters. As well as highlighting the slow pace of community developments, the report carried a second message: community care was beginning to develop in a skewed and distorted way.

The emphasis of the NHS seemed to be on the closure of the old hospitals or reductions in the number of hospital beds, rather than the provision of care for individuals in the community. It was evident that the move towards hospital closures and reductions in scale were driven by economic pressures rather than by the care plans of the chronically mentally ill or those people who had become long-stay hospital residents. The recommendations of the audit commission were both coherent and radical as they looked for a single agency to manage the funds currently divided between the health service and the social services' departments. In addition, they recognized that the responsibility of the NHS for the mentally ill did not stop at the decision to discharge long-stay patients. The report called for local 'champions of change' to take the lead in their organization; the emphasis was to be on action rather than rhetoric; local services should be integrated based on neighbourhoods; multidisciplinary working was encouraged; new partnerships were proposed between the statutory and voluntary sectors.

The report carried a great deal of weight as the Audit Commission was independent of both central and local government. The research evidence it produced supported the view that in the decade from the mid 1970s to the 1980s community care continued to owe more to ambition than achievement. What remained unsaid was even more interesting, however, as there was no attempt to clarify and articulate the form or content of the desired model of community care. Did care in the community mean a wholesale closure programme for the old hospitals, with resources being transferred to the neighbourhoods? Did community care mean the development of a range of complimentary services but run by separate agencies who were implored to coordinate their activities? Did community care mean handing over the responsibility for decision-making to a new body, as the existing agencies had demonstrably failed? Such questions hung in the air following the Audit Commission Report, but they provided a platform for the government to initiate an overall review of the management of health and welfare services both in community-based and institutional services.

The Griffiths Report of 1983 and the Audit Commission of 1986 were important preludes to the three major White Papers of the late 1980s. The three White Papers *Promoting Better Health* (1987), *Working for Patients* (1989) and *Caring for People* (1989) set the political and operational agendas for health care policy and practice for the remainder of the century. In order to understand the forces which shape mental health policy and practice in Britain at the end of the twentieth-century it is important to understand these papers and their implications for professionals and service-users alike.

*Promoting Better Health* was, in part, the result of a government consultation on health needs and priorities and it focused on primary health care services. At the heart of the paper was a reiteration of the view that there was a greater need to emphasize preventive health care and the prevention of diseases rather than the traditional emphasis on hospital services for acute conditions. The paper also contained a subtler message which sought to change the standing of patients from passive recipients of services to informed consumers. The aim of the White Paper was to improve the standards of health care overall by giving greater emphasis to primary health care, rather than the secondary or tertiary services of the district hospital or regional specialty. The aims as stated above seemed laudable and almost beyond question. However the way in which these approaches were to be implemented by central government led to anger and dissent within the general practitioners' professional organizations. The White Paper sought to introduce a new contract for general practitioners and dentists which set out annual targets. These included targets for annual health checks for all patients over 75 and 3-yearly checks for patients not seen within the period. One of the most contentious targets in the new contract was that set for vaccination and immunization which, especially for practices in inner cities, was regarded as difficult to achieve.

Despite bitter wrangles between the British Medical Association and Kenneth Clarke, Secretary of State for Health, (reminiscent of the 1946–1948 disputes) the issue was eventually settled in 1990, and the new contracts introduced. Ironically, the BMA, which had so vigorously opposed the passage of the parliamentary bill in 1946 introducing the NHS, appeared as the staunch defenders of the service 40 years on. The impact of the reformed general practitioner services had little or no effect on the availability or quality of services for the mentally ill. This was both curious and alarming as primary health care was one of the major routes into specialist mental health care and a key source of treatment itself.

The same was not to be true of the other two White Papers which appeared in 1989 as they were to have a profound effect on the organization, funding and approach to health and social care for all patients, including the mentally ill.

Central government again commissioned Sir Roy Griffiths, this time to look at the way community care services were organized and, in light of the Audit Commission report, make recommendations for change. Griffiths began work in 1987 and produced his report *Community Care: Agenda for Action* (1988). The Griffiths review was insightful and timely but part of the message contained in the report was to establish a greater role for local government. This was politically distasteful to the Conservative government and especially to the Prime Minister. Griffiths called for a clear policy on the development of community care services with adequate resources being made available to achieve this. The Griffiths Report, like the Audit Commission, did not set out either clear definitions of community care or the model of service which was preferred. Rather he looked to the criticisms of the existing arrangements and sought to address them. For example, he argued that if services were failing because they were piecemeal, then the solution was to look for comprehensive and integrated services in their place. He looked to 'packages of care' to be delivered to each individual in need, although the provider of component services could be one of a number of agencies.

Griffiths recognized that just as the range of people in need of community care was wide, then so the range of services needed to be wide in scope. Unlike much of traditional thinking in health and welfare planning, Griffiths sought to ensure that community and institutional care was not polarized; the Griffiths view was that community care applied to those in hospital as well as those currently living in local communities. The Report also sought to change the status of the person receiving care along the lines of the consumer model which was popular in government circles. The Report encouraged individuals to be actively involved in the planning of their own care programmes but he did not go on to suggest that health and social care should be managed or shaped by those who used those services. Griffiths did, however, give emphasis to the question of quality of service and he saw the gateway to improved quality as the setting of specific standards of care which could be monitored at the point of delivery. This idea proved to be one of the most attractive and robust approaches which emerged from the late 1980s review of the management of care.

### TOWARDS NEW LOCAL SERVICES

Other specific changes were also taking place which were to have a direct effect on the mentally ill during this period of intense official activity. The new Mental Health Act of 1983 has already been discussed and this was supplemented by the inclusion of the mentally ill in new legislation on disability. The Disabled Persons (Services, Consultation and Representation) Act 1986 updated the 1970 law and included explicit provision for the mentally ill. In particular, it required the Secretary of State for Health to provide information to parliament on the development of health and social services provision for people with a mental illness living in the community, as well as those receiving in-patient care. The first of these reports was made in 1990 and it described government policy on mental illness along the lines of the Audit Commission Report. In the view of the Secretary of State there were four main components of a proper, locally-based service:

1.  Provision for children and adolescents with psychological problems; these should be primarily community-based.
2.  Adequate services for assessment and treatment of adults who require short-term admission to hospital or longer-term treatment, including asylum.
3.  Sufficient places in hospital and local authority hostels, sheltered housing and other forms of accommodation for those needing residential care outside hospital along with adequate day and respite services.

4. Effective, coordinated arrangements between health and social services, primary health care teams and the voluntary sector for continuing support to the mentally ill.

Whilst these statements fail to describe either the overall model of service which informed government plans for community care or the practical way in which such services would be managed and monitored, it did go some way towards helping to understand the overall perceptions of central government on the provision of patient and client care.

Central to the Griffiths' argument was the criticism that much of care in the community was fragmented and uncoordinated. District health authorities and social services departments had developed uneven, uncoordinated and confusing patterns of provision, although they served the same localities. The Griffiths' solution to this central problem was to name Social Services Departments of the local authority as the lead agencies to manage and coordinate care in the community. Such a message was unwelcome by a government which had worked to reduce the role of the local authorities in other areas such as education and housing. The result was a delay of over 18 months in central government responding to the second Griffiths Report, with a White Paper which set out the intentions for new legislation on care in the community.

It was clear by the beginning of the 1990s that over a decade of uninterrupted Conservative government had produced no grand plan for social policy and welfare services. What did exist was an approach to issues which was common to all government thinking in the health and social care field. This approach rested on three key assumptions: first, seek to reduce the degree of reliance on the state as a sole provider of services; second, set out the broad aims of public policy without the detailed map on how to achieve these ends; third, look to the model of the market economy to introduce new, more business-like approaches to improve the efficacy and productivity of health and welfare resources. These three approaches of more self-reliance, centrally-directed strategy and a belief in the power of markets, were cornerstones of *Working for Patients* (1989) and *Caring for People* (1989). Between them these two White Papers set out government's thinking on the role and management of health and welfare services for the rest of the decade. On these papers and their implementation hung the future of the NHS and social services in Britain. It is these two papers and their implication which will now be examined in Chapter 5.

# 5

# The politics of working for patients

## REFORMING THE NATIONAL HEALTH SERVICE

*Working for patients* was published in 1989 as the prelude to legislation to transform the management of health care in Britain. The White Paper was the result of a year-long review set up by the Prime Minister, Margaret Thatcher. The review sought to examine the way the NHS was managed and funded; as there was concern within the cabinet as to the efficiency and responsiveness of the system established in 1948.

The ideas which resulted were radical and far-reaching as they sought to transform the NHS from a single organization at district level which identified priorities and provided services, into two distinct and separate functions of purchasers and providers of patient services. The very title of the White Paper hints at the extent of the change: instead of giving people what it was thought they wanted the reformed NHS would provide what was required. This seemingly simple idea masked a range of complex political, technical and ethical issues for politicians, professionals and the British public alike. It is important therefore to grasp what the White Paper actually said and to try to understand what followed from it. The transition from White Paper to legislation was, however, to prove to be stormy and testing for politicans and professionals alike. As a result of this process the final result of the White Paper had a rather different emphasis from the one envisaged at the outset.

Although it was unclear at the time of publication of the White Paper the period following was essentially one of negotiation and amendment. *Working for Patients* set out seven key changes in the way health care was organized and provided:

1.  Delegated decision-making was to be encouraged in order to make the service more responsive to the needs of patients.
2.  Two types of hospital would operate within the NHS, self-governing trusts and directly-managed units.
3.  New funding arrangements would be used on the principle that 'the money would follow the patient'. Therefore money would be able to cross traditional administrative boundaries.
4.  Additional medical consultant's posts would be created especially to reduce waiting lists for operations.
5.  General practitioners could become budget-holders in order to obtain a defined range of services from hospitals.
6.  New health authorities would be created at Regional, District and Family Practitioner levels to purchase services.
7.  Clinical audit would be introduced to improve the quality of service delivered.

The title of the report was *Working for Patients* and the central theme was putting the patient first, however the White Paper did not propose to establish a patient's charter or to hand over the control of services to elected bodies of consumers. The approach taken by the Conservative government was essentially threefold. First, introduce the market place to health care and use competition to drive down costs and push up standards. Second, change professional behaviour by establishing standards and workloads through contracts. Third, apply the business management methods of the most successful parts of the private sector to the largest employer in the public sector.

Over the 18 months which followed the publication of *Working for Patients*, the implications of the paper were explored and developed. What the White Paper sought to do was to break the mould of the NHS which had remained virtually intact for 40 years and look to business solutions to tackle the tension between ever-rising demand for health care and the ability to resource and manage operational services. The White Paper proposed that the traditional dual role of health districts as both purchasers and providers of services should end and these two functions should be formally separated. New District Health Authorities should take responsibility for identifying the health needs of their resident populations and purchase services accordingly. The services identified by the authorities could then be purchased from a range of providers including the local hospitals and health services which had previously been integrated in the old health authorities. The relationship between purchasers and providers would be set out in contracts for services which established the volume, quality and price of each specialty.

### THE RISE OF A CONTRACT CULTURE

The arrangements for health care after April 1991 would therefore involve a separation of functions and new formal relationships between purchasers and providers set out diagrammatically in Figure 5.1. These arrangements were

*The purchasers*

| | |
|---|---|
| 1. District Health Authorities | 3. Family Health Service Authorities |
| 2. Regional Health Authorities | 4. Budget Holding GP Practices |

*Contracts*

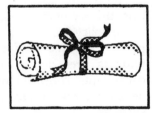

*The providers*

| | | |
|---|---|---|
| Directly-Managed Units | Self-Governing Trusts | Independent Sector |

**Figure 5.1** The contract relationship.

the normal way for commercial organizations to conduct their affairs but the approach, techniques and values were radically different from the traditional way of providing care within the NHS. The changes were even more dramatic, however, in their departure from the long-standing approach to health care provision, as the White Paper allowed for two types of organization on the provider side. The NHS had been based on the idea that local areas organized their health services to meet the needs of resident populations. The White Paper allowed for new 'self-governing trusts' to be established which were outside the control of the local health authority, albeit within the NHS. Those services which did not seek trust status remained under local control as 'directly-managed units', again within the NHS. The new trusts differed in other respects from the directly-managed units, especially in terms of their management board, which emphasized the business-like quality of the organization rather elected local representatives. The trusts also had greater latitude in arranging some of the financial aspects of their business, especially in raising capital monies to build or refurbish facilities which could generate income through contracts.

The organizational changes brought about by the White Paper clustered around four areas: the strategic management of the NHS, the idea of a market in health care, management of clinical resources and changes to the role of medical staff. These developments are summarized in Figure 5.2.

The White Paper was followed up with 11 additional papers from the Secretary of State for Health which added more detail to the policy framework of the original paper. These 11 working papers covered self-governing hospitals, contracts, GP budgets, prescribing, capital charges, medical audit, medical consultants' contracts, new health authorities, funding capital developments, education and training and information systems.

One of the issues raised by many critics of the White Paper was the fear of creating a two-tier health service which contrasted the trusts with the directly-managed units; by implication, the quality of health care available would depend on *where* it was sought. If such a claim could be sustained then this was likely to be a fundamental weakness in the new system after April 1991. Those who took this line, however,

NEW MANAGEMENT PROCESS

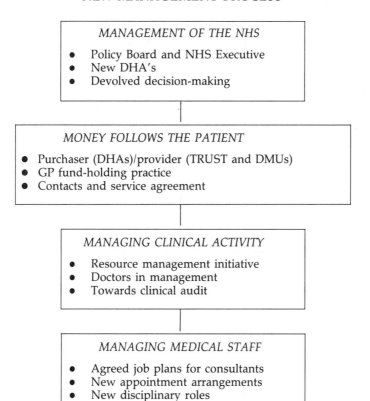

**MANAGEMENT OF THE NHS**

- Policy Board and NHS Executive
- New DHA's
- Devolved decision-making

**MONEY FOLLOWS THE PATIENT**

- Purchaser (DHAs)/provider (TRUST and DMUs)
- GP fund-holding practice
- Contacts and service agreement

**MANAGING CLINICAL ACTIVITY**

- Resource management initiative
- Doctors in management
- Towards clinical audit

**MANAGING MEDICAL STAFF**

- Agreed job plans for consultants
- New appointment arrangements
- New disciplinary roles

**Figure 5.2** Management issues in the NHS.

ignored the evidence of the long-standing divide in the NHS between teaching and non-teaching hospitals and districts. Since the eighteenth century teaching centres had been established in the inner cities in the large hospitals which provided easy geographical access to the greatest density of population. As a result of the drawn-out process of sub-urbanization, the inner-city population declined in absolute numbers. There was a marked increase in social deprivation for those people who shared neither the commercial wealth of the city or the earned income of those who commuted to work in the city. People who lived in inner cities had higher levels of morbidity than might be found elsewhere, and as such served the needs of the medical educators. One of the consequences of this schism in health arrangements was the emergence of an unequal allocation of resources to the teaching areas over those that were non-teaching. It may be the case that the White Paper eventually serves to reinforce the inequalities in resource allocation, but it needs to be recognized that the NHS had, since its inception been organized on a two-tier arrangement. One of the major challenges for the teaching hospitals in the new NHS will be to justify their likely higher costs and the numbers of medical staff and beds in use. There is a tension between the needs of the purchaser and provider of teaching hospitals, who will be driven by a contract culture which seeks lower unit costs and higher productivity as well as providing an agreed level of quality of patient care. The needs of the teaching function and adherence to contracts in a market economy are not necessarily compatible.

### 'THATCHERISM' AFTER THATCHER

Before the first of the changes in the NHS could be implemented there was a sudden change of leadership of the Conservative Party. Margaret Thatcher faced a challenge for the leadership towards the end of 1990 and the Conservative parliamentary Party was asked to choose between Thatcher and Michael Heseltine. Despite winning this first ballot the majority was not sufficient to ensure a clear victory and Thatcher then chose not to face three potential challengers in a second ballot. However the issue which brought about this situation was not health, despite the imminent changes which were to be implemented in the April of 1991. Margaret Thatcher lost support from within the Conservative Party because of the perceived failure of the 'poll tax' reforms which had replaced the domestic rates and her resistance to European economic union.

The leadership contest of the second ballot was between Michael Heseltine, the ex-Secretary of State for the Environment, Douglas Hurd, Foreign Secretary and John Major the Chancellor of the Exchequer. The ballot resulted in a victory for Major as the choice of the Conservative parliamentary party to take the place of Thatcher as Prime Minister. Therefore it was to John Major that the task fell of continuing the radical

Conservative tradition established by Margaret Thatcher a decade earlier. One of the first public statements made by Mr Major was about his desire to work to create a classless Britain in the next decade. This suggested that John Major's political sentiments were rooted in the 'one-nation' conservatism discussed earlier rather than the market-lead approach promoted by Margaret Thatcher.

These differences are not about personal whimsy or an obtuse point about political philosophy, rather they go to the heart of the relationship between the state and the individual and the degree to which public services should be provided. If John Major was concerned to ensure that a classless Britain was created then he could look to the health service as a barometer of social and regional inequalities. If he sought to continue with the Thatcherite tradition then the market place would separate out those services which were financially viable and those which should continue in the public sector free at the point of delivery.

The implementation of the health changes was to fall to William Waldegrave who had replaced Kenneth Clarke as Secretary of State for Health. *Working for Patients* concentrated on hospital services and the scope of family doctors to influence those services. It said little about community services or those for the chronically ill as this was the concern of the third of the government White Papers, *Caring for People*. It is this paper and the implications for the mentally ill which will now be considered.

## MANAGING HEALTH AND SOCIAL CARE IN THE COMMUNITY

*Caring for People* was published in November 1989 and it looked at the provision of community care for the 1990s and beyond. The White Paper's view of community services was one of a mixed economy of services in which state service was one partner amongst many. The White Paper was the mirror image of *Working for Patients* as it dealt with the provision of social care as well as health care. However, the pace of community care developments had been a concern of central government since the 1950s and it was a central issue in the 1975 White Paper on mental illness. To address this issue the 1989 document sought to clarify the roles and responsibilities of interested parties, disentangle the maze of financial support for community services and emphasize local decision-making. The underlying approach of the paper was to highlight community care as the service of choice for the majority of people in preference to hospital or residential care. The concept of community care had for so long been a convenient weapon in political polemic as it was thought of as both desirable and imprecise by both the political left and right. The government sought to clarify its own understanding on the issue in the following terms:

> Community care means providing the right level of intervention and support to enable people to achieve maximum independence and control over their own lives. For this aim to become a reality, the development of a wide range of services provided in a variety of settings is essential. These services form part of a spectrum of care, ranging from domiciliary support provided to people in their own homes, strengthened by the availability of respite care and day care for those with more intensive care needs, through sheltered housing, group homes and hostels where increasing levels of care are available, to residential care and nursing homes and long-stay hospital care for those whom other forms of care are no longer enough.
>
> *(Cmnd 849. p. 9)*

The White Paper was written with the knowledge of the demographic timebomb of Britain's ageing population, especially the accelerating numbers of people aged 75 years and over. It was argued that with over 6 million adults in the population with some physical, mental or sensory disability, the elderly and the disabled were a self-selecting priority group, especially as 4 million of these people were currently aged over 65 years. The government also identified the mentally handicapped as a priority group, especially as the number of specialist hospital beds had been halved to 30 000 since the beginning of the 1970s. The White Paper picked out the mentally ill for particular attention as 'the implementation of community care for people with a mental illness has given rise to particular concerns' (Cmnd 849. p. 13).

Before exploring the approach to the mentally ill in detail it is necessary to understand the overall objectives of the White Paper. There are six stated key objectives in *Caring for People*:

1.  To promote the development of domiciliary, day and respite services to enable people to live in their own homes whenever feasible and sensible.
2.  To ensure that service providers make practical support for carers a high priority.
3.  To make proper assessment of need and good case management the cornerstone of high quality care.
4.  To promote the development of a flourishing independent sector alongside good quality public services.
5.  To clarify the responsibilities of agencies and to make it easier to hold them to account for their performance.
6.  To secure better value for taxpayers' money by introducing a new funding structure for social care.

These six objectives seem attractive; a positive statement of the aims of community care provision. However, the objectives need to be considered in more detail as each has implications for professionals, carers, patients and clients alike. The first objective is to promote domiciliary, day and respite services, but by default does this mean that residential care becomes a service of last resort? The second objective is to provide practical support for carers; as the majority of carers in Britain are women does this mean that they are institutionally trapped in the role of carer without choice? The third objective is about assessment and case management, but whilst promoting case management as the 'cornerstone' of high quality care the White Paper fails to state which model of case management is preferred and why? The fourth objective is to promote the independent sector, although the White Paper fails to ask precisely what is meant by an 'enabling' role for social services? The fifth objective is to clarify the responsibilities of agencies in order to make them more accountable for their performance; what the objective fails to ask is whether such clarification is likely to lead to 'boundary' disputes between agencies? The last objective is to secure better value for the taxpayer through the reform of the funding arrangement for community care; in practice this concentrates on the shift of social security benefits away from residential care; it is unclear as to how this represents better value for money when the aim is to cut or transfer costs rather than promote choices between services. Perhaps one objective is to reduce public expenditure but this seems to be at odds with another objective – to promote a flourishing independent sector which would rely on public funds to pay for individual packages of care.

## THE HEALTH AND SOCIAL CARE DIVIDE

*Caring for People* talks about 'community care' as an amalgam of health care and social care, but lead responsibility for managing the changes was to rest with the local authority. Furthermore, their role was to change subtly, from being a traditional provider of services to that of an 'enabler' of services to be provided. New community care plans would be agreed between the health authorities and the local authority and new funding arrangements would be introduced to promote care in the community. In addition, there would be new forms of support for carers and the local authorities would be required to introduce formal assessment procedures and establish case management to reduce the fragmented provision of services. To achieve all of these changes it was essential that a new collaborative arrangement had to be created between health and social care services. In taking this view the White Paper attempted to set out the respective responsibilities of the two major agencies: health authorities and social services departments. These responsibilities are set out in Table 5.1.

The White Paper talks easily about the distinction between 'health needs' and 'social needs', but such contrasts imply that these things are somehow self-evident. Where for example, in the care of an elderly person with dementia, does the distinction come in providing for the burden felt by carers and relatives? The White Paper describes a world which is neat and conceptually tidy; in which health and social care agencies operate in a systematic way regulated by contracts and care plans. Such a world is unrecognizable to patients with mental illness, carers struggling to cope or to professionals trapped between the rising expectations for better managed services and the reality of under-funded and uncoordinated local provision. Much of the planning for mental health services is done in a political and service vacuum where innovation remains as untested proposals in unread planning reports, or as an unfulfilled wish-list for future services.

**Table 5.1** New health authority and social services department responsibilities

| Responsibilities | |
|---|---|
| *Health authorities* | *Social services departments* |
| Identify the health needs of the local population | Assess individual need and ensure delivery of packages of care |
| Ensure hospital discharge procedures are in place and agreed with local authority | Produce clear community care plans consistent with the health authorities |
| Experts for assessment | Independent sector |
| Prepare and agree joint community care plans | Establish 'arm's length' inspection and registration units for residential care |
| Provide continuous care for 'ill' people | Monitor the quality and cost-effectiveness of community care provision |
| Identify building and development sites with the private sector | Establish consumer feedback and complaints mechanism |

Butler (1991) argued that the central challenge offered by *Caring for People* is to find ways of recognizing the fragmented state of current services and doing something about it. To the patient or the client the niceties which distinguish the roles and responsibilities of health authorities from social services departments are obscure and remote; what they want is appropriate help now. The fragmented and uneven nature of health and social care services has resulted in people with mental illness becoming one of the most disadvantaged groups in society; they are promised comprehensive and seamless services on one hand and are subject to compulsory hospital treatment on the other. The problems facing mental health service-users and the response of the community care initiative will be examined next in Chapter 6.

# 6

# Managing change from the centre

*Caring for People* treats the mentally ill as a special case as it stated that there exists a justified concern for the availability of community services for people with a mental illness. This sentence casually expressed both a recognition of the failure of community care investments since 1975 and a belief in changing the way in which services are delivered. However, the document referred to two specific characteristics of services which it was claimed were the policies of successive governments after 1975; these two features were to encourage the development of locally-based services and for health, social services and the voluntary sector and private sector to work together to meet the needs of people of all ages. It is curious that the Mental Health Act 1983 did not set out to achieve this objective.

The White Paper argued that there are four components of a proper locally-based service for the mentally ill:

1. Community-based provision for children and adolescents with psychological problems, allowing access to hospital-based services.
2. Services for the assessment and treatment of adults whose conditions require short-term admission to hospital, and for the longer-term treatment, including asylum, of those for whom there is no realistic alternative.
3. The provision of sufficient places in hospital and local authority hostels, sheltered housing, supported lodgings

or other similar forms of provision for adults with a mental illness needing residential care outside hospital, together with an adequate range of day and respite services.

4.  Effective coordinated arrangements between health and social service authorities, primary health care teams and voluntary agencies for continuing health and social care of people with a mental illness living in their own homes or in residential facilities. These should include suitable domiciliary services, support to carers, and the training and education of staff working in the community. (*Cmnd 849. p. 55*)

At a casual glance these descriptions of the major components of a 'proper' locally-based service appear to be rational, progressive and humane; however, such important claims need closer scrutiny. Whilst the emphasis on assessment and treatment for adults is laudable it is specifically limited to those who are thought to require short-term admission to hospital, this begs the question as to why the same degree of attention is not available to the majority of mentally ill patients who are treated in the community? The statement goes on to describe the need for asylum, especially for those for whom there is no realistic alternative. What is not explained is on what grounds are services thought to be realistic; is it a technical judgement or one based on cost? For those people thought to need residential care the emphasis in the paper is on beds and their classification rather than the way in which individual needs are assessed and provided for; again the emphasis is on the patient's relationship to hospital. The last of the four components of these proper, locally-based services concerned the effective coordination of health, social services and the independent sector; What is significant is the absence of the key central government departments such as the Benefits Agency which holds responsibility for income maintenance and the Department of the Environment which controls decisions on the funding of public sector housing.

## HOSPITAL VERSUS COMMUNITY CARE

The White Paper claims that these policies became possible because of research and clinical experience which showed what was possible outside the long-stay hospital. Whilst this claim is not remarkable, there is no one single piece of empirical evidence presented to support such a claim. Where are the references to the research?; if the evidence is so compelling why does the paper give such a degree of emphasis to the minority of patients who receive in-patient services in hospital. There *is* good evidence to show that the great majority of people who present with mental health problems can be, and are treated without having to be separated from their own homes and communities, but it is not presented or examined in the White Paper. Mosher (1983) looked at the evidence from research on alternatives to hospital care. She cites 37 separate studies comparing non-hospital with in-patient psychiatric treatment which found the former to be as good or better than the latter in outcomes for the patient, as well as being cheaper. Mosher develops the argument a stage further by referring to the literature review carried out by Kiesler (1982) which looked at psychiatrically disturbed people randomly allocated to mental hospitals and community forms of care. The conclusion reached from the review was that those patients admitted to hospital were more likely to be re-admitted than those people treated in alternative ways, despite there being no clinical differences between the two groups.

The potential change envisaged by the White Paper for the mentally ill is considerable as it provides for a new form of relationship between agencies and those who receive their services as well as between themselves. But what is the likely impact to be on individuals who have pressing mental health needs now. Open almost any social services department's case notes or health service patient's records and sad, tragic and confusing personal histories come spilling out. Such records may contain a case summary as follows:

Catherine Ambler is a 46-year-old woman who lives with her husband and two teenage daughters in their own home in a suburb at the edge of the city. She has cared for her elderly mother for the last 7 years since her father died suddenly. She works during term time as a cleaner in a local school, but she has been on sick leave for the past 5 weeks with pain in her lower back. Her GP, Dr Ericks, has not been able to find anything specifically wrong with her back, but he is concerned with recent changes in her appearance which has become shabby. Mrs Ambler agreed to allow her husband Jimmy to make a joint appointment to see Dr Ericks. This resulted in Jimmy describing the increasing 'bad moods' his wife has and the fact that their two daughters now stay with friends during the week. Jimmy Ambler wants 'something done about his wife's mother and some tablets to stop his wife's back pain'. Dr Ericks referred Mrs Ambler to a local Consultant Psychiatrist to see 'if he could sort this one out'.

For Mrs Ambler, Jimmy and Dr Ericks the boundaries between 'health' and 'social' care have little real meaning; they are not interested in the arcane differences between health service and social services' responsibilities. What they want is help now with problems which seem to be intractable: Mrs Ambler wants the worry of her dependent mother to be sorted out as well as a cure for her increasing lack of energy and painful back. Jimmy Ambler wants his wife to be the person she once was and for their two daughters to spend time with them as a family. Dr Ericks wants to break the increasingly desperate cycle of surgery visits by the Amblers for whom he has no instant solution. This story of the Amblers and Dr Ericks is a piece of fiction, but there are many such people trying to find their way through the complex maze of health and welfare provision each day. Some of these people are referred to specialist services but many struggle along in desperation with their problems, feeling that the system of health and welfare has little to offer them.

The discussion which followed the publication of *Caring for People* included a rich mixture of fantasy, anxiety and good sense. One of the myths of the community care changes is that the world of health and social care would be turned upside down on 1 April 1991 with the implementation of the changes. However, in July 1990, the then Secretary of State for Health, Kenneth Clarke, made it clear that the original government timetable for implementation was to be varied. The major parts of the community care changes were shelved until 1993 and only the changes for the mentally ill were to be implemented in April 1991 as originally envisaged. Central government blamed the local authorities for not being prepared in time to implement the changes and the local authority associations blamed the government for slowing down the process because of a preoccupation with the size of poll tax bills. The net effect of this change was that for at least a 2-year period the new arrangements for community care provision for the elderly, physically and mentally handicapped was to be suspended. Ironically, during this period it was to be administratively easier to find public funding for a place in a private residential home than to make available domiciliary support to allow a person to remain in their own home with support.

## NEW MONEY AND OLD PROBLEMS

The government did announce in circular *HC(90)24* the arrangements for the new specific care grant for the mentally ill which was to be made available from April 1991. This allowed for a new discretionary grant to social services, to improve the social care available to people with a mental illness in need of specialist psychiatric care. This Specific Care Grant was not available to individuals who used mental health services as such, but to social services as an agency. The money made available by the Department of Health was passed to the Regional Health Authorities who triggered payments to the local authority social services department. These arrangements made no formal provision for a role for the new purchasing District Health Authorities or the provider, directly-managed units or self-governing trusts. Their involvement was dependent on the attitude of the lcoal authority, despite it being a requirement of the grant that there must be prior agreement between health and social services about the kind of social care provided. This arrangement was all the more confusing as it was already a prime condition of the grant that it was targeted at patients and clients already involved with a specialist psychiatric service. This was an important condition, as it placed considerable limits on the voluntary organizations who could use the grants, as they had to have the support of both health and social services. In effect, this meant that the grant could not be used to fund services which were radical alternatives to the current providers of care or services. The grant did, however, allow for people who had psychiatric needs but who were not in touch with current services to be helped; especial emphasis was given to the homeless mentally ill by the Department of Health.

The grant was available as revenue funding for 3 years initially and it could not be used for capital projects. In the

the first year 1991/92 the total monies made available nationally was £30 million, of which the local authorities had to find one-third. Unless the local authorities could show that they could achieve this 30% contribution they were ineligible for the new monies. In a period where the collection of the new poll tax was proving to be particularly difficult, the local authorities faced two pressing problems. First, many authorities (especially those in the inner city areas) faced reduced income as a result of non-payment of poll tax. Second, for those who were poll tax capped by central government there was little or no prospect of raising their contribution when unable to maintain existing services. If the local authority decided to match their 30% contribution to the government's 70%, they then had to come to an agreement with the District Health Authorities and the new Family Health Service Authorities on the specific schemes to be funded. Once a formal agreement had been reached and the Regional Health Authority had been notified, the new monies could be released by central government to the local authority. In this arrangement the Regional Health Authority does not act in an inspection or monitoring role but rather as a postbox for the funds passing between central and local government.

One of the key problems with the specific care grant initiative was the amount of money available. An allocation of £21 million from central government, topped up by another £7 million from the local authorities divided between the 100-plus social services departments made for very limited new spending. The formula used for the allocation of monies, the Personal Social Services Standard Spending Assessment (PSSSSA) resulted in what appeared to be anomalies. Manchester Social Services received an allocation of £240 000 whilst Berkshire had £270 000, as did Devon (because of the simple per capita formula used to allocate resources rather than any assessment of need).

Resources for people with mental illness represents only a marginal part of the overall social services' expenditure, when compared to other services such as children and the elderly. The Specific Care Grant continued the same theme and served to reinforce the place of mental health services as a minor activity of the social services departments. Whilst the small allocations of additional marginal monies were welcomed they were insufficient to alter either the organization of mental health care or the processes which were developed. In short, the Specific Care Grants were unlikely to make a significant difference to service quality or the life-chance for people with mental health problems as they served only to fund change at the margins.

### THE LOCAL CONSEQUENCES OF CENTRAL PLANS

The planned changes in health and social care are talked of as if the world of need, provision and services would change fundamentally from 1 April 1991 for the mentally ill, and from April 1993 for other groups in need of community care. The overall relationship between the state and the individual in receipt of health and social care services has changed as a result of the White Papers and the subsequent legislation. These changes are, however, the first instalment of a series of changes which move care from a demand basis to a mixed economy of marketed services. Figure 6.1 reiterates the main changes prompted by the three White Papers.

These changes are the start of a new process of continued change although it is likely to prove to be easier to make changes in the organizational structure of department and agencies than in the attitudes of those people who work in them. By and large the people who manage and provide services under the Community Care Act 1990 are going to be those who worked in the fragmented services which the legislation set out to change. What will change in the first instance is the responsibilities of those professionals working in health and social care and the expectations of those who seek care in the community. It is perhaps easier to think about changes to the hierarchy of agencies than about changing the attitudes of those people who work in care agencies. This is especially so when the myth of the 'right' structure is so powerful in organizational thinking. It is commonly believed that there is such a thing as the right structure for all organizations and it is only a matter of time and continual re-organization before the solution is reached. This approach, which has been so dominant in many health and social care agencies, avoids the key issues of agreeing common visions of the service to be provided and ensuring that there is agreement about the end product. Once this has been achieved it

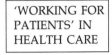

'WORKING FOR PATIENTS' IN HEALTH CARE

- GPs to purchase some services
- DHA purchaser
- DHA assess needs
- £ follows patient
- Capital charges

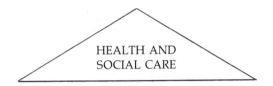

HEALTH AND SOCIAL CARE

'CARING FOR PEOPLE' IN THE COMMUNITY

'PROMOTING BETTER HEALTH' IN PRIMARY CARE

- Local authority lead role
- Local authority to 'enable' services
- Jointly agreed community care plans
- Support for domiciliary care
- Collaboration with health and independent sector

- New GP contracts
- Information and choice for patients
- New standards of care
- FHSA new role

**Figure 6.1** White Paper changes.

is then possible to explore the ways in which services are provided.

DEMAND VERSUS NEED

If the objective of change in mental health services is to provide integrated, comprehensive and effective services then the starting point is to examine what is meant by these three concepts and establish who subscribes to this view. Many agencies and organizations have shining examples of good practice, but they are often isolated or hidden from the mainstream work of the department, separated from the management process. There is much to be learnt for the mentally ill and other groups from those people who are recognized by service-users as providers of excellence. This does not mean that the shape or structure of the organization is unimportant; the point is that it should follow from the purpose of the agency as form follows function. What is more important is the attitudes of professionals who represent those agencies to clients, patients, carers and the new purchasers.

The Community Care Act 1990 brings together health authorities and social services departments in order to agree on two types of community care plans. The first is strategic and to do with the overall direction and pace of service provision; the second is the plan of the specific care provided to a known individual. There is, however, within this arrangement an inherent difficulty which stems from the way that the two agencies traditionally see the world. For over 40 years health service planning has been shaped by a public health view of the world which focuses on epidemiology to help to understand local needs. In contrast, the social services departments created in the 1970s have been dominated by a social work view of the world rather than a wider social services' perspective. In particular, needs have been seen in terms of social casework whereby they are absolutely unique and individual to the particular client. All too often the sad reality has been that in both health and social services 'need' has not been looked at from the same perspective. For the NHS it is often the needs of a general population and for social services it is the specific needs of an individual. Both agencies also suffer from the understandable confusion which is made between 'need' and 'demand', which often results in the continued provision of an existing service when an alternative may be more appropriate and effective. One of the most powerful aspects of the new community care legislation is that it forces social policy issues back on to the centre stage of the political agenda rather than as a minor character in the wings.

*Promoting Better Health, Working for Patients* and *Caring for People* share five common policy and operational threads:

1.  the separation of the purchaser and provider function;
2.  the use of contracts for services;
3.  recognition of the need to listen to those who receive services;
4.  the rise of a mixed economy in health and social care;

5.  a more business-like approach to service management.

However, the reform of health and social care generates a number of potential obstacles to the successful implementation of the new approach. There is no easy way to find agreement on the scale of health and social need as the world does not naturally divide in to such a neat scheme. This is especially so when so many of the discussions and negotiations are conducted in an information vacuum. If it is possible to find a way of assessing need then it is likely that this will produce a volume of demand for services which prove to be outside the scope of current resources. The separation of the purchaser and the provider function, which is at the heart of the changes, is not as simple as it might initially appear: the distinction between health needs and social need is blurred and inexact. If the community care plans are intended to ensure a closer working relationship between agencies to promote a better quality of life for clients and patients then how can we tell when this has been achieved? This is a theme which will be explored in more detail in Chapter 9, in looking at the alternatives to the traditional ways of planning overall services and providing for the needs of individuals. The stated intention of the new legislation is to enable health and social services to work more closely together; however there is a widespread belief that traditional joint planning has failed other than as a device to administer the marginal monies of joint finance. The short-falls of joint planning arrangement will be explored in Chapter 8, in looking at new relationships between those who purchase, provide and depend on mental health services.

Throughout the White Papers and the government literature on changes in community services there is a great deal of emphasis given to the role of the case manager. Much is expected of case management to overcome the traditional fragmentation of services experienced by clients and patients alike. But there are difficulties in reaching common understandings on what is meant by case managment. It is the central role of case management which will be examined in the rest of this chapter.

## CASE MANAGEMENT: THE NEW PANACEA?

Case management is central to the view of service organization and delivery within *Caring for People*, although increasingly the official literature refers to 'care management' as a more personal term than case management. There are a number of assumptions made in the White Paper which also have a significant bearing on the style and effectiveness of care management. Care management is seen primarily as the responsibility of social services departments although latitude is provided for people from a variety of professional backgrounds to take on the role. Three further publications by the Department of Health/Social Service Inspectorate (1991) sought to develop a more complete explanation of the implementation process of care management assessment. Care management and assessment are described as follows:

> ... one integrated process for identifying and addressing the needs of individuals within available resources, recognising that those needs are unique to the individuals concerned. For this reason, care management and assessment emphasise adapting services to needs rather than fitting people into existing services, and dealing with the needs of individuals as a whole rather than assessing needs separately for different services.
>
> *DoH/SSI (1991), p. 7*

Care management is described as a process which consists of seven distinct stages:

1. Publishing information for prospective users and carers on the role of the care agencies and services offered.
2. Following referral information is collected to clarify the type of assessment required.
3. A practitioner is allocated to assess the needs of the client and carer in light of their circumstances and the local context of a variety of agencies being involved.
4. The practitioner works with the user in order to agree a care plan taking into account the full range of resources available locally.
5. The care plan is implemented in this stage by bringing together the range of financial and service resources required and negotiations begin with providers to make available a service.
6. A process of continuous monitoring is introduced following

the implementation of the care plan and the commitment of resources. The purpose of this stage is to enable the practitioner and the user to alter and vary the services in order to meet the agreed objectives.

7. At agreed periods the implementation of the care plan is formally reviewed with user, carers and service providers to ensure that the service and the plan continue to be appropriate and to assess the capacity for continued improvement.

The official view of the Department of Health is that most of the seven tasks set out above can be undertaken by an individual care manager, although it is acknowledged that they may be shared by different practitioners. This poses some difficulties in that the care manager is charged with taking a 'needs' view rather than fitting patients/clients into existing services. However, needs is defined by the Department as:

> ... the requirements of individuals to enable them to achieve, maintain or restore an acceptable level of social independence or quality of life, as defined by the particular care agency or authority. Need is a dynamic concept, the definition of which will vary over time in accordance with: changes in national legislation, changes in local policy, the availability of resources, the pattern of local demand.
>
> *DoH/SSI (1991), p. 10*

This definition significantly weakens both the concept of a needs-lead service and makes ambiguous the role of the care manager. Rather than establish criteria and a process for the assessment of objective and subjective needs, the approach taken by the Department reinforces the inequalities in health and social care which already exist, by tempering the definition of needs to fit into the resources available. For the care manager in such a situation, the problems of reconciling assessment of needs and the allocation of scarce resources creates an impossible strain. Whilst this dilemma is essentially organizational and to do with the inability of the agencies to discharge their responsibilities; in practice it becomes the personal responsibility of the care manager.

### THE PROBLEM OF ASSESSMENT

The 'assessor' function in the care management process as set out by the Department is essentially that of the covert gatekeeper. This person distinguishes between those people who look for help and those who receive it. The role of the gatekeeper is to ration service provision and to re-direct others to more appropriate agencies. The assessment of individual needs in the terms of the community care provision is a statutory duty of the local authority. After April 1993 the local authority will be duty-bound by the NHS and Community Care Act 1990 to coordinate arrangements for the multi-agency assessment of community care needs. The care manager's role only comes into play once the person has been formally referred to social services and it is agreed that public funds should be spent to meet their assessed needs. The White Paper recognized that people's needs change over time and therefore need to be monitored. However the care manager is only brought into play 'where an individual's needs are complex or significant levels of resources are involved' (Cmnd 849. p. 21). What the document does not say is that all individuals's needs are complex to them, nor does it define what is meant by the term 'significant resources'. In the latter part of the financial year even relatively modest sums could be regarded as significant to an overspending department. The stated responsibility of the case manager is to ensure that the needs of an individual are regularly reviewed, resources are managed effectively and that each service-user has a single point of contact.

*Caring for People* outlines five elements of effective case management based on pilot projects in Kent, Gateshead and Durham Social Services Departments:

1. Identification of people in need, including systems of referral.
2. Assessment of care needs.
3. Planning and securing the delivery of care.
4. Monitoring the quality of care provided.
5. Review of client needs.

*(Cmnd 849. p. 21)*

The paper makes clear that it is not essential in the Department's view that the case manager actually carries out all of these tasks personally, rather the role is to ensure that they are completed by identified personnel. Many of these tasks would have been recognizable to traditional case workers who pre-dated the creation of the generic social services departments. The point is well made in an unpublished paper sponsored by the American National Institute on Alcohol Abuse and Alcoholism:

> people from many disciplines within the human service field have performed the functions of linking the needs of the individual with the appropriate resources in the community, and of helping people become more independent and functional. Providers of these services have included hospital social workers, child protection workers, probation and parole officers, welfare workers, drug and alcohol counsellors, and community mental health workers, amongst others.
>
> *Willenbring et al. (1990)*

There are as many models of case and care management as there are settings for the delivery of care. Clifford and Craig (1989) identified four models which were likely to be adopted in Britain in the late 1980s and the 1990s:

1. The first of these was based on the multi-disciplinary teams within health districts which developed 'key-workers' into case managers. In the view of Clifford and Craig such a team would be led by a senior clinician such as a consultant psychiatrist who would manage the budget.
2. The second form of case management was again within the health service, but it was in addition to existing teams within districts. The role was seen as coordinating the services of specialists.
3. The third model was based on the social services department which 'bought in' services as required for each individual client as part of the separation of the purchaser and provider function within social care.
4. The fourth of the approaches was the consortium model which was the most radical departure from the traditional provider arrangements. In the new arrangement both health and the social services would surrender budget control to a new joint agency which would be staffed by professionals and non-professionals alike.

The attempts by Clifford and Craig to classify and order the varied approaches to case management is a useful but strictly limited starting point. Curiously the first model based in the health service automatically assumed that the medical consultant was the appropriate person to act as the case manager, although no medical skills were required for the role. In the second model the assumption was made that the case managers 'would be CPNs or largely non-professional staff' thereby implying in one simple phrase that community psychiatric nurses were not professional and that case management did not require much more than the coordination of existing services. The third model whereby the social services enabled or bought in services as required fails to discuss the relationship between the purchasing and provider function, let alone the setting and monitoring of standards. The fourth model, the consortium, was the most radical departure from existing practice. The writers failed, however, to discuss the idea or the implications of jointly-managed services which seemed to offer interesting opportunities to break the log-jam of fragmented services which were evident by the beginning of the 1990s.

Shepherd (1990) looked specifically at the role of the case manager in services for people with long-term mental illness and attempted to identify the relative advantages and disadvantages for the successful coordination of care. Shepherd is more questioning of the issue of who should be the case manager and what kind of training is likely to be required to carry out the role successfully. Shepherd concluded that case management has the potential to coordinate care effectively but it is not an alternative to a comprehensive range of services for the mentally ill. He makes the telling point that the need for coordination of effort is greater in the community as opposed to the relatively closed world of the hospital institution. Shepherd noted that the data on the effectiveness of case management is both weak and contradictory and there is much to be done in providing a better knowledge-base to test the outcomes of case management.

The work of Research and Development for Psychiatry (RDP), the London-based research group, has stimulated some of the most interesting ideas on community care in the early 1990s. They led the development of case management through the introduction of eight projects on six sites in Bromsgrove, Hastings, Nottingham, Guy's and Lewisham, Leicester and Cambridge using Department of Health monies. Ryan, Ford and Clifford (1991) produced a report for RDP which traced the emergence of case management and community care policies in Britain. They contrast and compare case management, care management and the care programme approach in terms of six functions which are: defining the client, assessment, developing the care plan, introducing packages of care, provision of a direct service and monitoring and review. Their conclusion is succinct and clear:

> There are however some striking differences. To begin with, both the care programme and case management can perhaps best be seen as overarching organisational processes. As such, their main task is to ensure that the functions of assessment, care planning, monitoring and review are undertaken. Only in case management, however, is one named person explicitly involved in the whole process from assessment to review; only in case management is the same person also involved in direct work with the client.
>
> *Ryan et al. (1991), p. 35*

One of the core problems of care or case management is the relationship of the purchaser and provider functions. If assessment and a formal eligibility criteria are used to act as a means of gatekeeping to ration service uptake, then the care manager is effectively a *provider* of service. Paradoxically the result may be that following assessment the client may not receive a service. If the care manager is not part of the assessment process, but holds the budget for services independently of other practitioners, then he/she is a *purchaser* of services who awards contracts on an agency basis and coordinates resources on behalf of the service-user.

Despite the relatively long history of the role of the case manager and the recent appearance of the title there are a number of key unresolved tensions implicit in the task as envisaged by the White Paper. The decision to admit an individual to have access to the resources of the social services department will not be the task of the case manager, as it will fall to the gate-keeping assessor. However there is an issue as to whether the case manager has a devolved budget in a particular department. If not, then how will they ensure that the appropriate set of resources are released to meet the client's assessed needs? If the case manager is a budget holder then they will feel the annual pressure of departmental rationing and resource management irrespective of the identified needs of the clients. One of the most pressing areas of service need in the mental illness field is in the arrangements for the planned discharge of patients from psychiatric hospital back to the community. Despite this being a statutory duty of the local authority under section 117 of the Mental Health Act, it appears from the annual reports of the Mental Health Act Commissioners that it is infrequently observed adequately. Case management as envisaged in a discussion paper by the *NHS Training Authority* (1990) identifies four key features of case management which could meet the needs of patients coming out of psychiatric hospitals:

1. To ensure a voice and choice for the individual consumer.
2. To resolve specific problems of crossing boundaries where various agencies are involved.
3. To resolve difficulties in interweaving statutory and informal care and to strengthen natural support to the individual from family, friends and other members of the community.
4. To ensure that resources are used effectively and efficiently to achieve the above on behalf of the individual consumer.

Perhaps the NHS Training Authority picture of the specific mission of the case manager is rather widespread and idealized but there is no doubting the accuracy of the targets.

## THE CASE MANAGER'S DILEMMA

The case manager will have to grapple with the labyrinth of social and health care and find a niche within the social services as a parent organization, whilst acting with an independent view. This is likely to prove very difficult for an individual to cope with unless there are a number of safeguards built in to the system. These could include a formal process of professional audit for specific services with agreed outcome measures as well as a service which is driven by individual care plans for clients. It is also going to be essential that the case manager operates in a political climate which is supportive of the role for example with agreement from the local authority elected members and the health purchasers and providers.

One of the central difficulties which the case manager is likely to experience is the new function of the social services department as an 'enabler' of service provision rather than as a direct provider. In practice this is likely to be an area for conflict when care packages are constructed which include significant funded services from the voluntary and private sectors.

There may also be a tension for the case manager who has to juggle with a range of professional and moral concepts within the assessment process; notably, how will the individual professional find a balance between the patient's/client's risk, entitlement and dependency and the personal responsibility of the case manager. Perhaps all this process will do is to make explicit the tensions and shortfalls which are deeply embedded in the current system and professionals will cope with these issues as before.

The financial aspects of the provision of care in the community are complex, bordering on the bewildering. Benefits Agency funds can be provided for residential care for people in independent homes with additional money from income support and housing benefit. The public funds allocated from central government through the revenue support grant will have to be rationed in policy terms by the elected members. Specialist funding for particular groups such as the mentally ill and the specific care grant, joint finance projects and income from charges will also have to be utilized appropriately. Finally for a large part of the population who continue to live in their own homes there will be social security income through the income maintenance system. In order to ensure that clients who live in the community or in the residential sector maximize income and those funds are used correctly, the case manager will have to develop an acute financial acumen to master a system which was previously characterized for its complexity.

The case manager is an innovative solution to the problem of fragmented care services provided by a number of agencies. However, the case manager's role is the fulcrum of the reformed system of care in the community as the task is to bring together social and health care services to meet the assessed needs of individual patients and clients. Much rests, therefore, on the shoulders of the individual case managers, especially given that there is no clear description of the relationships with either their own agency or service-users. *The central role of the case manager is to reduce the fragmentation of services for individuals in need; despite being part of the same system which produced those incoherent, confusing and uncoordinated services.* The case manager has to address the two key problems of health and welfare services, first these services have shown themselves historically to be weak at ensuring continuity of care and, second, individual service-users have never been stakeholders in services to the degree that they had an effective voice in decision-making.

Following the publication of *Caring for People* the Department of Health set about filling in some of the missing details which would inform operational services in health and social care. In particular the Department published circular *HC(90)23* which set out ideas on the 'Care Programme Approach' for the mentally ill. This paper was both revealing and contradictory. The official guidance from central government to District Health Authorities is set within the broad framework of the White Paper of 1975 but there is a note of caution as the comment is made that:

> ... providing adequate arrangements for the community care and treatment of some patients has proved more difficult and resource intensive than expected. In practice adequate arrangements have not always been achieved.
> *HC(90)23*

There is a view amongst those who have experienced attempts to resettle people from institutions to the community that adequate arrangements have rarely been achieved because of three obstacles. First, the paucity of resources available, not only to reproduce the facilities of the old hospital but also to meet the comprehensive needs of the individual. Second, the need to fund two services simultaneously, the declining old hospitals and the new community facilities, from a budget which is only capable of meeting one set of requirements. Third, the wholesale lack of coordinated services scattered amongst a range of agencies working in the same locality. The acid test for the new policies is the degree to which they radically tackle the well-understood problems of the existing services.

The care programme approach was intended for mentally ill people who are in touch with specialist psychiatric services. It was stated that local arrangements were to be negotiated between the relevant health and social services departments but the care programme would have three core elements:

1. Systematic arrangements for assessing health care needs of patients who could, potentially, be treated in the community as well as the regular review of those already receiving treatment in the community.
2. Systematic arrangements agreed with social services for assessing and reviewing social care to enable such patients to benefit from treatment in the community.
3. Effective systems for ensuring that agreed health and social care services are provided to those patients being treated in the community.

The approach emphasized the need for good interprofessional working and the involvement of patients and carers in discussions about the care programme. However, the care programme approach is a significant step back from the case manager as the key actor in the reformed provision for the mentally ill. In place of the case manager the government guidelines identified the 'key worker' as a pivotal figure. The stated role of this person is to 'keep in touch with the patient and monitor that the agreed health and social care is given'. The executive role of the case manager as a controller of resources and a person who services the client is missing.

At the outset of the reforms of health and social care services for people with mental illness in the mid-1980s, the key questions concerned the performance of health and social services agencies. The changes which ensued did not tackle these organizations as such, but rather their respective roles. By the beginning of the 1990s the alternatives were further diluted with the introduction of the key worker as a partial substitute for the case manager. The care programme approach is essentially a pragmatic response to the problem of funding the changes in health and social care with the emphasis being on reforms within existing resources. What is described is not a radical departure in either policy or practice, but rather a reiteration of the principles of good practice which were commonplace within many health and social services agencies. What is missing in the care programme approach is an honest appreciation of the politics of health and social care reforms. The issue which is avoided is the prospect of a significant increase in public spending which would result from switching the provision of services from 'demand' for what already existed to 'need' based on individual assessment and goal plans agreed with patients/clients. In place of this, the advice was to name one worker in each case as the key person and put the onus on them to communicate, monitor and review the provision of services to individual users. Such a development was a significant step backwards from the rhetoric of consumer choice which was heralded in the health and social care White Papers which preceded the care programme approach.

Like many of the health and social services reforms of the late 1980s and 1990s the separation of the purchaser and provider functions, case management and the idea of consumer choice were essentially imports from the American health and social care industry. Chapter 7 will examine the state of American health care and in particular the developments of services for the mentally ill. There are a number of reasons for looking at the American experience, especially the importance of the market as a mechanism to regulate health care and the development of services for the mentally ill within a free enterprise society. Such an examination may help to understand some of the sources of the health and social care reforms in Britain as well as providing an opportunity for policy and service comparisons between two differing societies.

# 7

# Mental health care in the United States of America

THE COMING CRISIS OF HEALTH CARE IN AMERICA

The key changes in British health care during the period of 'Thatcherism' resulted from a deep-seated belief in the ability of the market place both to reflect peoples needs and to meet them. Such a view was based on a vision of individuals solving their own problems rather than relying on the state to do so for them. The argument was taken further in the 1980s as the state and past governments were often characterized as interfering with the market and hindering competition which, in turn, restricted consumer choice. Thatcher and her economic and social policies were matched in America with the election of the Reagan administration which took an equally pro-market view of the world. Thatcher and Reagan shared a belief that the market was capable of regulating all aspects of life including health care. It was through the introduction of market forces in health care that the patient as consumer was thought to be best served. Equally, Thatcher and Reagan saw the solution to monopolistic suppliers and cartels in health care as being the 'de-regulation' of the health care industry, be it in the public or the private sector. Whilst Thatcher and Reagan shared a common set of beliefs, it was Thatcher who looked to the American health care industry as a model on which to base the reforms of the NHS, with the key principles of separate purchasers and providers, contract-based services and change through competition for markets. Paradoxically, as Britain looked to America for an alternative way of managing the

NHS, so the American health care industry moved deeper into financial crisis. The result was that as Britain sought to develop a market-based health service, America moved towards a state-funded system as a result of a deepening health care crisis.

Health care in America is a product of American society and as such it shares all of the strengths and weaknesses of that society. It would be misleading to talk of a 'system' of health care in America as there is nothing systematic about either the policy or the provision of health care. It is the very lack of any cohesive policies or comprehensive provision which is one of its hallmarks. It is these features, and others, which prompt commentators to characterize health care as being in crisis and in need of urgent reform. This chapter will discuss the state of American health care in general and look at the position of services for the mentally ill in particular. The purpose of this examination is not to eulogize or denigrate the services of a society which differs from Britain, but to try to understand how that society has tried to tackle similar problems to those found in Britain in the organization of health care.

Many of the changes in health care introduced in Britain by the Thatcher government found their origins in American health provision. American health care, like American society at large relied upon the market place as the central organizing principle to bring together those who had needs with those who sought to satisfy them. From this approach there emerged a series of ideas which have found their way into the NHS reforms. There are two central ideas which appear in *Working for Patients* and *Caring for People*; the separation of the purchaser and provider function, the use of contracts for services to regulate service volumes, price and quality.

The source of the coming crisis in American health care is money; in particular, the problems of rising costs for care and a growing reluctance to fund services by both the public and private sectors. The American approach to managing health care differs markedly from that taken in Britain since 1948.

The traditional approach of the NHS has been to ensure that a service is virtually free to all at the point of delivery. This means that the health service is funded by central government using revenue gathered from personal taxation and national insurance contributions. Since the late 1970s the proportion of personal contributions made for specific services has increased, especially for prescriptions of medication, spectacles and dental care. The basic assumption, however, has remained the same throughout five decades: services are available to all irrespective of their ability to pay. In practice there is a dual system in operation in Britain, whereby a small but developing private sector has emerged, usually based on an insurance or membership arrangement to fund services. In many NHS hospitals there are examples of private services using public facilities for a fee, usually with a higher standard of 'hotel' services for the patient.

The American approach, by contrast, has a long history of separate purchasers and providers of services with large insurance organizations such as Blue Cross and Blue Shield providing cover for a premium and buying in services from providers as required. In addition to this private arrangement for health care there is a public system of funding health provision in the Medicare system. This is funded by the Federal government and is regarded by many Americans as a last resort. For many Americans the cost of funding health care for themselves and their dependents is becoming a matter of major concern. Whereas it was common in the 1970s and 1980s for employers to offer packages of remuneration to their staff including health insurance, this has become the source of bitter dispute throughout the early 1990s. Some of the old industries such as iron and steel have contracted substantially during this period, but they still have to support the many people who have retired from the industry with relatively low-cost health cover. Some of this is provided by employers and some by the trades unions but increasingly they are unable to fund the cost of a larger, dependent, retired labour-force from a diminishing industrial base.

What is the scale and the source of these rising costs and the coming crisis of the Amnerican health care industry? The *Harvard Economic Review* (1989) estimated that despite a real decline in the funding for Medicare and Medicaid, 12% of American gross national product was spent on health care. This is in contrast to the estimated 6% of gross national product spent in Britain on health care. The article predicted that up to 1 000 hospitals could close by the end of the 1990s as many of them are inner-city charitable institutions which have been technically bankrupt for some years already. In circumstances where costs are rising and quality is declining the market mechanism leads to almost inevitable contraction in the numbers of viable providers. For those old hospitals which are already uneconomic there is little opportunity to modernize and compete in a market driven by rising costs. For the purchasers of health care, the insurance companies and the employers there is increased pressure to scrutinize and control costs. Over and above this there are an estimated 37 million Americans who are not covered by health insurance or whose cover is grossly inadequate to meet their needs. For these people life is increasingly precarious; illness and treatment present as a major fear.

## THE SEARCH FOR ALTERNATIVE FUNDING

As Britain looked to America for a model of health care in the late 1980s so Americans looked to Britain and Canada for alternatives to their own arrangements. Both Britain and Canada with its social insurance funding can accurately be characterized as 'systems of healthcare', whereas this is not true for the American approach. Individual Americans organize their health care either by negotiating it as part of a package of rewards at work, by buying it personally from an insurance company or by falling back on the partial provision of Medicare. Despite the growing importance of health as a social policy and political issue, it did not figure in the 1989 presidential elections. On the contrary, George Bush was actually elected on an explicit programme to curb any tax increases, despite the growing acknowledgement of the inability of many Americans to access or pay for health care.

American health care faced seven major problems by the beginning of the 1990s which reinforce the view that there is a coming crisis:

1. The growing reluctance of purchasers to fund the rising cost in health care.
2. A shortage of skilled clinical staff, especially nurses, due to a decline in the birthrate.
3. An emphasis on health provision for acute services which led to the under-development of services for chronic care.

4. An increasing health and social care challenge posed by the growth of an ageing population with the 'greying of America'.
5. The unknown costs associated with HIV and AIDS.
6. The cost of providing for health and social care arising from common catastrophic injuries such as car accidents.
7. The increasing cost of successful litigation and the medical insurance associated with it.

The impact of these pressures has been profound as health care is a key talking point in American public life, although as yet it has to surface as a political issue in its own right. There is much discussion as to whether access to health care is a right or a privilege and, depending on the point of view, the alternatives become more or less attractive.

Throughout the late 1980s and early 1990s the real impact of rising health costs was felt by the administrators and managers who were responsible for the operational running of health care services. The pressures on managers came both from the purchasers of care, who wanted to ensure value for money for their health dollar, and from providers who sought to protect the professional judgements and the quality of patient care. By way of response, the managers developed two strategies. First, they examined high-cost hospital admissions as well as developing new forms of service such as ambulatory care. Second, they sought to gather information to make comparisons between hospitals on both quality of care and costs to the purchaser. Once again the belief was that the well-informed consumer could shape the future of health care through purchasing decisions taken in the health care market. To understand how such an approach could work it is necessary to look in more detail at the operation of services in America.

## MANAGING COSTS AND MANAGING CARE

A number of innovative schemes were established in separate states across America, including Washington state, Iowa, Maryland and California. One of the most comprehensive was the Pennsylvania Healthcare Cost Containment Council (HC4) reported broadly in the British health literature by Butler (1990).

This statutory body was set up in 1985 with a brief look at three specific issues: to analyse escalating health costs, to look at ways of linking cost and quality; and how to provide wider access to health care regardless of the ability to pay. The Council consisted of 21 member agencies including Pennsylvania's business sector, labour organizations, state government offices, insurance companies, universities, health providers and consumer groups. The HC4 organization was based in the state capital, Harrisburg, with a permanent staff of 17 people. Early on in the project the principal mechanism for controlling costs was agreed: competition between providers, through the collection, analysis and distribution of standardized data on cost and quality, for all hospitals in the Commonwealth of Pennsylvania. It was argued that access to such information would improve decision-making on the purchase of health services and facilitate provision at an affordable price. The information produced by HC4 was used principally by three different groups: purchasers of health care such as Blue Cross/Blue Shield insurers; competitive providers working in the same field; and patients who wished to make informed choices about the services they used and paid for.

*The First Hospital Effectiveness Report* (Health Care Cost Containment Council, 1989) reviewed the 55 most commonly used Diagnostic Related Groups (DRGs). These were clusters of medical conditions which had a degree of 'family' resemblance and could be usefully drawn together from the thousands of detailed diagnoses available. By selecting these 55 it was found that over half of all hospital discharges would be captured in the data set. HC4 were then able to look at each hospital in turn and analyse the average degree of sickness, measured in a standardized way, within the first 2 days following admission. The types of indicators used were vital life signs with weighting to indicate the patient's ability to respond to treatment. Medical outcome information on the success of each treatment within a specific DRG was also included. The HC4 staff produced data which were intended to help clinicians, referrers, purchasers and patients to compare hospital performance and costs.

The HC4 reports allowed for comparisons to be made in Pennsylvania between hospitals' costs, utilization of resources, severity of condition and morbidity by DRG. The first findings

revealed wide discrepancies between hospitals on the relationship between cost and performance for the same set of patient
problems. In one hospital 42 cases of a particular procedure
resulted in a cost of $3008 per case, whereas another hospital
with 31 cases in the same DRG charged $5051 per patient for
the same procedure. Even though the cost differed by $2000
per patient the average severity was the same, as were the
outcomes, measured by mortality and morbidity. There are
a number of possible reasons for the wide variation of cost
despite the same outcomes: overall case mix of patients,
teaching commitments, higher local living costs, percentage
of free care provided on a charitable basis, nursing levels,
capital costs and the numbers of Medicare patients paying a
lower rate. But what is undeniable is that there is an appetite
for such information and a growing expectation that health
care professionals, clinicians and managers, will increasingly
be held publicly accountable for the cost and quality of their
services.

The Cost Containment Council's work can be used as an
educational tool to turn the focus of health care professionals
from hospital output to patient outcomes. The data set could
be used to negotiate a prospective payments arrangement to
underpin contracts between purchasers and providers. As
Britain looks to America for ideas on the management of health
care, so the American approach still appears to be a collection
of services with no over-riding organizing principle, other than
the market place. What the HC4 approach brings to the debates
on the organization of health care is a belief in the rational
use of good quality information to enable service-users to
choose between providers on the basis of their performance.
Other American states have developed other alternatives to
understanding the demand for health care and the cost of
providing it. Foremost amongst these is Oregon which has
created a form of cost–benefit analysis to try to understand
the balance between resources spent and the quality of life
derived. In the Oregon case the emphasis is on explicit
rationing of services through a priorities exercise. Both Pennsylvania and Oregon face the same philosophical dilemma, 'is
health care a right or a privilege?'

Whilst these approaches are innovative in themselves, they
are not adequate substitutes for the social policy and political

debate on health care. Such a debate would ask what type of health care system does a particular society want?; how does it intend to pay for it? It is just such a debate which has emerged in Britain in the early 1990s as a result of the government reforms. From the Westminster viewpoint this may have been one of the unintended consequences of the reform programme.

The work of HC4 said nothing about services for the mentally ill and there are a number of good reasons for this decision. Provision for the mentally ill has a separate history to the mainstream of American health care and the approaches developed elsewhere are not always applicable to the mentally ill. There are, for example, Diagnostic Related Groups which refer to the mentally ill, but their usefulness is more restricted than among some other patient groups. In the HC4 approach, diagnosis was used as a proxy for predicting outcomes, but this is a poor indicator of outcome for cases of mental illness. This is particularly so as there are many other influential factors which determine outcome, some of which are medical and some social. One of the particular features of the 55 DRGs chosen by the HC4 team was that over half of all patients treated fell into this small cluster of acute services. For the mentally ill, life as a patient or ex-patient of mental illness services is often chronic in duration. It is simply not possible to record absolute outcomes in the same way as for a patient undergoing a surgical procedure. The rate of change for the mental patient may be slow and hesitant, with occasional setbacks. The road to recovery involves every aspect of an indivdual's life including their home circumstances, relationships, employment prospects, self-esteem as well as the impact on health professionals.

To understand more about the development of services for the mentally ill in America and their possible impact on services in Britain it is necessary to look at the emergence of policy and provision within an American context. Such an approach may clarify our understanding of changes and innovation in American mental health services and in turn lead to a reappraisal of the constraints and potential for good practice in Britain.

The coming crisis of American health care is already well advanced as there are medical institutions which have failed economically; there is a growing unwillingness by purchasers to meet the escalating costs of medical care and a significant part of the population is already disconnected from health care services. In such a crisis-ridden situation, how do the mentally ill fair? There is no single source of evidence on which to form a clear opinion on this question.

This approach allows us to look at two key issues. First, the relationship between clinical activity and cost. Second, the relative performance of a range of providers. This approach may prove to be of more use than trying to find some generalized explanation for the policies and practices of a society as diverse as the United States of America.

THE SEARCH FOR A SYSTEM: CHANGE AND CONTINUITY

Washington DC in the early 1990s presents the visitor with stark contrasts and conflicting images of life in the capital city of the richest society on earth. As well as being the seat of government and the political centre of power, Washington is home to large numbers of homeless and mentally ill people who live on the streets and exist at the very margins of society. Visitors to the State Department are confronted by people begging for small change or sleeping out in public parks. Areas close to the city centre which are quickly developing into fashionable and artistic neighbourhoods, such as Dupont Circle and Adams Morgan, are also the homes for the poorest, most destitute and disturbed Washington citizens, whose membership of society is at best tenuous and at worst non-existent. How could such a situation have developed in a society which only three decades earlier waged a 'war on poverty' and sought to develop mental health services in the community? In order to answer this question it is necessary to look further at the development of American mental health policy and to distinguish between the political rhetoric of reform and the actual experience of service-users.

Rothman (1985) reviewed the development of mental health policy and provision in America from the early part of the nineteenth century to the Second World War. He traced the emergence of the asylum in the nineteenth century and changes to the state mental hospital in the twentieth century. Despite the change in title and approach, Rothman argued that he was writing about the 'enduring asylum', as the key function of custodial care for the chronic patients remained the same. Rothman's argument suggests that not only did the custodial asylum survive a number of attempts at social reform but it both endured and as a result stifled the emergence of mental health services in the community. The push for reform and change focused on the mental hygiene movement who sought to bring mental illness in to the public health area, with care outside the exclusive asylums and state hospitals. Rothman identified one of the key sources of resistance to change as the attitudes of the leading professionals within the state hospitals who were responsible for the management of the institutions. He points to the fact that between 1880 and 1940 the numbers of people detained in the mental hospitals grew more than five times faster than the general population. Talbott (1978) takes a rather different view from Rothman as he referred not to the enduring asylum but to the 'death of the asylum'. Talbott argued that change had occurred to a significant degree and this was influenced by the particular circumstances of individual hospitals; policy changes applied to the institutions, changes in the pattern of service delivery and wider changes in social attitudes towards the mentally ill.

Goldman, Morrissey and Klerman (1985) sought to explain changes in American mental health care in terms of 'cycles of institutional reform'. This analysis took the Worcester state Hospital in Massachusetts as a model for the American experience of mental health care. Morrissey *et al.* argued that this single hospital accurately mirrored the cyclical pattern of reform and setback of the institutional care of the mentally ill in America. The changes in provision for the mentally ill are charted from the initial creation of small therapeutic asylums in the early nineteenth century to the large, cheap and impersonal warehouses established by the end of the last century. The response in the latter part of the twentieth century to the problems generated by these institutions has been, it is argued the re-emergence of local community services whose primary function is therapeutic rather than custodial. This ebb and flow of change and resistance is traced for the Worcester State Hospital as a paradigm for the provision for the mentally ill in America.

Somewhere between Rothman's notion of the 'enduring asylum' and Morrissey *et al.*'s explanation of the 'cycle of institutional reform' lies the experience of the user of services for the mentally ill. Ironically, the early history of American mental health provision reflected so much of the experience of their British colonial masters whose own asylums were described in Chapter 1. Much of the effort of those working and living with the state mental hospitals was directed at the development of alternative types of service which enabled the mentally ill to live as part of communities rather than apart from them. So many of the debates on mental health policy and provision in Britain find an earlier echo in the American experience. Two such different societies seem to have so much in common in providing services for the mentally ill and, in particular, in attempting to take corrective action to set right the effects of past policies.

Butler and Thomas (1990) looked briefly at the development of community-based mental health services in America and drew attention to the part played by developments in forms of treatment which emerged after the end of the war. Notable amongst these developments was Kaplan's crisis theory which stressed the importance of brief therapeutic interventions for people in acute crisis, the rapid assessment and management of soldiers suffering acute stress reactions from warfare and the technological developments in medication for acute psychosis in the 1950s. These changes in professional practice allowed for the possibility of patients to be returned rapidly to their communities as an alternative to a prolonged stay in the state mental hospital.

These developments were mirrored by a new-found energy and enthusiasm within government to look for alternatives to the state mental hospitals for the provision of services to the mentally ill. However, what is unclear is what drove the movement away from the belief in institutional care towards alternative forms of provision in the community. There are a number of factors which have emerged, albeit in a fragmented and often incoherent form. There appear to be five key factors for the new enthusiasm for provision in the community:

1. **Economics:** it was thought to be cheaper to provide services in the community.

2. **Demand:** service-users sought legal protection from detention in the state hospital.
3. **Viability:** many institutions proved unable to sustain either acceptable standards or costs for care.
4. **Alternatives:** new forms of private care emerged to compete with the large institutions.
5. **Scandal:** the isolated asylums were historically associated with maltreatment and abuse.

THE PROMISE OF COMMUNITY MENTAL HEALTH SERVICES

At the beginning of the 1960s, as Britain was implementing the new Mental Health Act and the critical review of hospital provision, the American government was responding to the first of a series of papers which sought to change mental health provision fundamentally. In 1961 a Joint Commission on health, education and welfare, published *Action for Mental Health*. This paper set out proposals for the creation of Community Mental Health Clinics specifically to reduce the need for prolonged or repeated hospital care. This type of service was seen as part of an overall range of services including general hospitals with integrated psychiatric units and separate hospitals for the chronically mentally ill. The ideas of the 1961 paper were translated into legislation in the Community Mental Health Act 1965, which sought to establish new Community Mental Health Centres (CMHCs). However, their remit was such that they were set up as panaceas for most mental health problems. Jones (1988) argued that the five essential elements of the CMHCs; in-patient care, out-patient services, partial hospitalization, emergency services and consultation and education were fraught with practical difficulties. Jones identified lack of clarity for geographical boundaries; professional isolation resulting from role-blurring, the ensuing growth in conservatism of those not involved and 'burn-out' of overworked staff. The initial interest in the CMHCs was considerable but this did not translate itself into the predicted growth of centres nationwide.

In the original 1961 plan it was proposed that CMHCs should be established for every 50 000 people. In all, federal funding was eventually provided for just over 700 separate CMHCs across America and these provided access to services for just over half the total population. Goldman, Adams and Taube (1983) established that out-patient attendances increased from 1.5 million to almost 2.5 million over the three decades from 1950 to 1980. However, over the same period the population of the state mental hospitals fell from over 0.5 million to 0.12 million, a decrease of 75%. Goldman and Morrissey (1985) analysed the increased numbers attending out-patient clinics and observed that this was a different population to those previously involved in mental health services. The new recipients of psychiatric services were not people with acute psychosis or the chronically mentally ill, but the 'worried well'.

Throughout the 1970s and 1980s in America there was a marked shift in the way in which mental health services were provided. Following on from the creation of the CMHCs there was a parallel development of the run down of the old asylums and the state hospitals, ranging from overall reductions in the numbers of patients to wholesale closures of individual institutions. The rationale for these changes was said to be the new policy of provision in the community but the economic argument to save money seems to have been at least as strong. The CMHCs were established but not in the numbers or locations originally envisaged by the 1965 legislation. So what happened to the hundreds of thousands of people who were previously long-stay patients of the old state hospitals? These former residents of the hospitals became the first casualties of the community care policy which was incomplete and open to wide interpretation. The CMHCs were funded by the Federal government and the money wholly bypassed the state hospitals, but the new community centres did not reproduce the full range of services previously offered by the old hospitals. The attraction of the CMHCs was that they offered services to the mentally ill in the community without the stigma associated with the old state hospitals. The CMHCs failed, however, to ensure that the most basic of human needs, shelter, was available to those who received services. Despite their relative isolation from mainstream society the state hospitals did provide shelter, food, clothing, companionship and recreation for the long-stay patients. Whilst the move towards community provision was undoubtedly a positive development in social policy for the mentally ill, in practice the new form of provision did not meet the range of needs of the mentally ill in the community. One of the key results of these shortfalls was a drift by large numbers of chronically mentally ill people into the inner cities. Some people found their way into other forms of institutional care such as private nursing homes where, by 1980 there were 700 000 residents. Others joined the ranks of the homeless or ended up in the prison system. By the beginning of the 1980s the association between the chronically mentally ill and the rising numbers of homeless people was well-established in the major cities of America. In time, a similar picture was to appear in the inner cities of Britain.

Some CMHCs which emerged in the 1970s and which continue to flourish in the 1990s provide sophisticated services and a range of care for the local population. One example is the Mental Health Centre of Boulder County, Inc., in Colorado. This organization provides, on behalf of Boulder County a comprehensive service to the acute and chronically mentally ill of a total population of 200 000 people. The catchment area includes the wealthy university town of Boulder, the semi-industrial city of Longmont and a range of small settlements and communities between Denver and the Rocky mountains. In such a setting the CMHC has worked together with the agencies of state, county and city government to develop a range of services, from preventive programmes for child abuse to clubhouses for the chronically mentally ill. One of the key characteristics of the approach developed in Boulder is the degree to which the development of services have been managed. This has been achieved through partnerships between agencies and governed by contracts specifying patient volumes, service quality and price. Each element of the Boulder system is, in effect, a separate enterprise linked through the management structure and the commitment to developing the Centre. In each of the Centres, contracts, patient numbers, quality standards and cost for service are all endorsements of the system from the patients and carers. It is perhaps possible to see why the Boulder CMHC has thrived when so many of those established in the cities have failed. There has been clear and consistent leadership over a sustained period; the area is attractive to staff, the lifestyle for patients is less hostile than many other places and the political support from government and the other agencies has proven to be robust.

For many people the CMHCs had failed only 15 years after their introduction as they had rejected any responsibility for the care of the chronically mentally ill who did not have access to funding by the health insurance companies. The chances of a person with a mental illness having access to an appropriate range of services became an accident of geography and it was clear that mental health services were not part of a system of health and social care. Other than the rhetoric of the federal government there was no clear policy or provision to ensure that coordinated services were available to the chronically mentally ill either in times of crisis or to provide the continued support to sustain people in the community. Jones (1988) pointed out that the Mental Health Systems Act 1980 introduced case management as a means to overcome some of the shortcomings mentioned above, but at the same time these changes gave greater emphasis to the judgements of professionals rather than to the expressed needs of the consumers of the services.

## INNOVATION IN SERVICES FOR THE CHRONICALLY MENTALLY ILL

By the beginning of the 1980s it was clear to professionals and politicians alike that there was a need to break the log-jam in American mental health policy and provision. It is interesting to note that this move towards a more concerted and coherent service was inititated in services aimed at those people with chronic and enduring mental health problems, rather than those people with minor psychological problems. Services for the long-term mentally ill which had traditionally been the poor relation in health care, became the setting for some of the most innovative developments in mental health care. The repercussions of these developments have yet to be felt in other parts of America and within services for other groups of people with mental illness. What the innovative services working with the chronically mentally ill developed was a new way of formulating the relationship between a range of agencies and of deploying resources on the patients' behalf. It is these innovative services which will be discussed in the rest of this chapter.

The initial efforts to deal with the shortcomings of existing provision focused on the delivery of services; the best known work in this field is that of the federally-funded National Institute of Mental Health (NIMH), which looked to support innovative projects in the substance abuse field. The most comprehensive and innovative development in services for the chronically mentally ill was taken by the Robert Wood Johnson Foundation (RWJF), a philanthropic arm of the Johnson and Johnson Company. The RWJF had a long-standing record of funding initiatives for the homeless in America and this was the means by which the plight of the long-term mentally ill came to their attention. In so many of the cases they were involved with there was both a homelessness problem and an unaddressed mental illness issue. They looked at examples of good practice in the mid-1980s in such places as Dane County, Wisconsin and the Massachusetts Mental Health Care Centre in Boston and identified a number of features which seemed to be important. Shore and Cohen (1990) identified three key features as follows:

1.  A comprehensive range of services and programmes ensuring appropriate care for persons at various stages of illness and disability.
2.  Assignment of clearly defined and continuous responsibility for each client with chronic mental illness, whether in hospital or the community.
3.  Budgetary control over all relevant services and settings, with fiscal incentives for providing appropriate and cost-effective care.

In short, what Shore and Cohen described was a patient-centred system of health and social care for the chronically mentally ill which encouraged and rewarded innovative good practice between professions.

In 1985 the RWJF established a new programmme on chronic mental illness which provided financial and other help to nine American cities, specifically to help the very people who had been forgotten in the move from state hospital provision to the CMHCs. The RWJF spent a year beforehand researching the issue and as a result made a significant discovery which was to influence powerfully the future of the project. Miles Shore, Director of the project described this as follows:

A year of intensive research revealed that most problems in delivering care to persons with chronic mental illness was due not to the nature of the available services, but rather to a lack of organized systems of care.

*Shore and Cohen (1990), p.1212*

This not only acted as a critical starting point for a new way of perceiving services for the mentally ill but it also served to lead the pilot projects away from traditional forms of organization. The point was made earlier that the emphasis of the CMHC approach was on the delivery of care to individuals in specific communities. The starting point of the RWJF approach was not on the delivery of care but on the organization of systems of care. When the emphasis was on the delivery of care it tended to reinforce the boundary demarcations between agencies and fuel the fragmentation of services. The RWJF approach was essentially about the integration of services and providers into a single system specially intended to tackle head on the problem of fragmented services. In their initial review of existing provision and service organization the RWJF looked at the number of interested parties with separate and uncoordinated responsibilities for the mentally ill. In particular they emphasized the multi-layered political machinery involved from the state, county and city authorities as well as the geographical separation through different boundaries and the range of funding agencies who provided welfare, housing and support services. At the heart of the RWJF approach was a belief that the only radical way to address the quality and availability of services for the chronically mentally ill was to seek a new alliance for radical change in service management and organization. The way in which they went about this was to attach a number of conditions to the grant aid on offer and to invite applications for pilot site status. The key condition was an assurance of commitment from the political leadership at state, county and city level to the creation of a new centralized authority to manage the services for the chronically mentally ill in the area. This new authority would have responsibility for all mental health services, both hospital-based and in the community. In all there were five conditions put on the grant monies: to create a central authority responsible for clinical, administrative and financial tasks; to ensure continuity of care; to develop a full range of services; to establish a housing plan; to seek out new sources of finance. The grants were available to the 60 American cities with populations over 250 000, and in all applications were received from 56 of these.

## INTEGRATED CARE FOR MENTAL HEALTH

In 1986 nine cities were awarded the RWJF grants in Austin, Texas; Baltimore, Maryland; Charlotte, North Carolina; Cincinnati, Columbus and Toledo, Ohio (as one entry); Denver, Colorado; Honolulu, Hawaii; Philadelphia, Pennyslvania. The expressed purpose of these grants was to change the existing system of provision and purchasing of care within the cities backed up by the political support already agreed as a condition of the grant application. In a society where the basis of health care is the purchase of a service for a fee there has been a long-standing tension between the funding of services and the ability to pay. This is especially marked in the case of the chronically mentally ill who are in the worst possible position to purchase services. Not only are they unable to meet the actual cost of health care, but they also may not be able to establish an address in order to access existing services. The RWJF approach sought to cut through these difficulties by not tinkering with the detail of the delivery of services but by trying to establish a single coherent system of mental health care which was capable of meeting the full range of needs of the individual coping with chronic mental illness.

In all, the RWJF provided a total of $29 million cumulatively to the nine cities, including a low-interest housing development loan over 5 years. Housing was a vital element of the project given the experience of the CMHCs and the evidence of the association of chronic mental illness and homelessness. As a result, a joint initiative was established with the federally-funded Department of Housing and Urban Development (HUD) which provided 125 Section 8 rent subsidies to each of the cities in the pilot project.

What benefit has the approach been to service-users and professionals alike and how were RWJF to judge the degree of systems change achieved? The demonstration site in Columbus, Ohio for example was established with the support of the local County Mental Health Board and it had as its objective the creation of a client-centred treatment system delivered by continuous treatment teams. These five teams provided outreach, primary treatment and specialist provision for people with dual diagnosis of functional psychosis and substance abuse.

Part of the project was a formal commitment to an evaluation carried out during the 5-year life of the nine demonstration sites. This task was contracted to the University of Maryland, Mental Health Policy Studies Programme who carried out an independent evaluation of the projects. In particular the evaluation sought to capture two distinct features of the pilot schemes: first, to describe the process of implementation of the programme and, second, to establish the impact on the lives of clients of the projects. Goldman et al (1990a) described the work as an evaluation which evolved into a programme of research. There were five key areas of study in the evaluation: individual sites; community care, housing, finance, and disability and vocational rehabilitation. The evaluation began with an attempt to articulate the relationship between the various elements of the centralized authority, this 'logic model' gave an account of the new structures, improved processes and specific outcomes for individuals with chronic mental illness. One of the key findings of the evaluation is likely to be that progress may be uneven and out of step with what was expected. The picture of the development of a specific project may vary in practice from that which was envisaged at the outset; for example, improvements may be made for individual clients but not for their immediate carers.

Goldman, Morrissey and Ridgely (1990b) reported their interim findings of the evaluation of the site studies of the RWJF programme. In particular, they focused their attention on the creation of the centralized authority established to give leadership to services and to reduce the fragmentation of services for the chronically mentally ill. Their initial findings reiterated the original approach of the RWJF project which regarded the centralized authority as 'a promising strategy and not a proven intervention'. The creation of the centralized authority in each city proved to be more demanding and time-consuming than had originally been believed. Not all of the sites had achieved a degree of control over state-run facilities such as the mental hospitals. Even where such control exists the timetable to complete the process is likely to be greater than originally thought. The involvement of the RWJF undoubtedly meant that additional resources became available, where otherwise this would not have been the case. In particular, new access to subsidized housing for the chronically mentally ill has been a significant feature of the projects, just as they were missing from the CMHC developments of the 1960s and 1970s. Perhaps the most significant achievement of the RWJF demonstration projects is that they have managed to bring the chronically mentally ill centre stage in local political thinking in nine major American cities. By doing so they have achieved a commitment to seek radical change in the quality of life for these clients by recognizing that their needs are only met by a range of services working in common purpose with a shared agenda for change.

The RWJF approach is not without its critics and Rosenberger (1990) argued that the idea of a central organizing authority is politically flawed for many of the same reasons which dogged the CMHCs. He argued that the idea of the centralized authority involved the existing agencies giving up voluntarily some of their power and authority. If this is to be achieved, Rosenberger argued it has to be seen as a political rather than an organizational problem. Likewise, the solution is not organizational but political.

The RWJF approach does have a number of features which need to be highlighted as examples of innovation, good management and professional practice. The central feature of the approach is the commitment to dealing organizationally with the problem of fragmented services as both service planning and car delivery are jointly recognized as the responsibility of the new, centralized mental health authorities. This approach is based not on a set of directives or prescriptions which are mechanically applied to a specific area. Rather they are a working method which allows local practice to develop out of the direct experience of local service-users and professionals. Neither is the approach dominated by one single ideology or powerful professional interest group. The commitment to producing a coordinated service for the chronically mentally ill within the RWJF demonstration sites is one which requires agreement by all levels in the mental health services from the individual user, the professional, the senior managers and the politicans. Perhaps at the heart of the RWJF approach is a set of values which is often despised elsewhere or dismissed as rhetoric. The values suggest that if those people who believe in their ability to develop a quality service are supported financially and politically, better services for clients and professionals can be established which are also more cost-effective.

The RWJF demonstration sites do focus on something which is essentially appealing to Americans of all political persuasion in that it is about providing opportunities for individuals working together to prove their potential. The RWJF sites seek to offer choice to service-users and professionals alike.

LESSONS FOR BRITAIN FROM THE AMERICAN EXPERIENCE

The RWJF-funded demonstration projects, in contrast to the CMHCs, looked to the new central authorities and case management as ways of dealing with the fragmented services for the chronically mentally ill in the inner cities. In one of the Baltimore projects, for example, each client is allocated a case manager to establish an agreed care plan between the agencies and the client. Problems are identified using the SHARES approach (Symptoms, Housing, Activities of daily living, Recreation, Employment and Significant other such as family). This approach was devised by Stein and Test (1980) in their original work in Wisconsin. The role of the case manager is rather like that of a key worker in that she/he devises a care plan with the client. However by way of contrast with the keyworker the case manager has overall responsibility to ensure the plan is implemented by others. Case managers act as advocates and service coordinators in this approach and the client is therefore less likely to become wholly dependent on one individual for the delivery of services. This is a real risk of a system of services which invests all responsibility in a single keyworker who may, in the client's eyes, be both the purchaser and provider of services. Such an arrangement is fragile and wholly dependent on the keyworker who may be moved or leave the agency at short notice, thereby cutting off the flow of services to the client. There are some interesting parallels with the care programme approach which is being introduced in Britain in the early 1990s and which was discussed in the last chapter.

There is no room for complacency when comparing the situation in Britain to that of America. In the decade up to 1987 the number of hospital residents in Britain fell by 30% from 84 000 to 60 000. Over the same period the Department of Health (1989c) reported that the number of residential places in the community increased by only 4000 places. This was despite a situation where the numbers of officially homeless people was increasing and the growth of 'cardboard city' within walking distance of the Palace of Westminster provided the only home for disturbed and chronically mentally ill people. Britain also saw a rise in the prison population to one of the highest per capita in Europe with overcrowding of Victorian gaols and unrest appearing as routine features of life for people at the margins of society. By the beginning of the 1990s there was a growing acceptance that many people who found their way into the prison system had serious mental health problems and hospitals, gaols and the street were increasingly alternative forms of disposal for the mad, bad and the destitute. Those people who had links with mental health services often found these bounds to be tenuous and strained: the developing approach of managed care through the introduction of care plans or case management did not operate outside the boundaries of the health or social services catchment areas.

## POLITICS, RESOURCES AND PRACTICE

Towell and Thomas (1989) looked at the lessons from America in light of the publication of *Caring for People* and their review of services for people with learning difficulties. It is interesting to note the number of similarities between the organizational problems for mental health services and for those for people with learning difficulties. Towell and Thomas argued that in order to have a positive impact, the White Paper changes needed to incorporate long-term development strategies which are both visionary and responsive. They emphasized the need for incentives for change and the time required to enable wholesale systems change to mature. In noting the existence of a mixed economy of care in America they highlighted the need to develop the role of 'enabler' for traditional providers of service and the creation of a 'provider market' to allow a range of services to develop. In their visits to areas as diverse as Arizona, Massachusetts, Mitchigan, Minnesota and Nebraska they recognized the same characteristics as the RWJF sites, notably the key role of political support from the agencies and the central organizing role of the case managers.

In his review of the effectiveness of case management for mentally ill people, Huxley (1990) looked at 14 case studies of case management systems. He argues that there needs to be a separate and new model of care developed for the chronically ill rather than the adaptation of models drawn from services for acute patients. Huxley highlights the range of different models of case management rather than assuming that case management itself is a single approach or solution to a range of problems. This point is directly connected to the degree of effectiveness of case management itself in Huxley's view, as the more successful programmes in the study were those which were specific about their objectives. Furthermore, the more successful programmes clarified the model of case management to be used and were specific about their target group. In this sense the degree of effectiveness achieved by the case management systems reviewed in the study was directly related to their claim not to be universal panaceas.

Many of the problems being faced by patients, clients and professionals alike, in Britain, bear a remarkable similarity to the American experience, especially in living with fragmented services. This is despite the differences in approach and attitude between the two cultures and the existence of a system of health and social care in Britain which is absent in America. Many of the features described above are specifically American and are the product of specific local circumstances, although there is much which can be adopted by service purchasers and providers in Britain. However excellent, the detail of specific services cannot be mechanically transferred to the situation in Britain in the early 1990s. Mental health and social care services in Britain must find local solutions to problems which will work within the particular social, cultural and political context. It is this issue of developing, managing and delivering mental health services which will be considered next in Chapter 8.

# 8

# Mental health services in the inner city

MANCHESTER: DEVELOPMENT AND DEPRIVATION

This chapter is different from others in this book in that it is an attempt to describe and examine a particular mental health service and the impact of the NHS and community care reforms. It is a less tidy process than describing policy changes and organizational re-structuring as it is dynamic and changing. Many of the issues discussed below are partially developed as there is a necessary degree of experimentation and testing in introducing change. However at the same time a service has to continue to be provided to people referred to the department. This chapter is essentially a case study of a process which is only partially complete. It is an attempt to record some of the issues, approaches and ideas which have resulted from change imposed from outside such as the White Papers and some change which has been generated from within, such as changes in the way services are managed. To those who are looking for a simple recipe which can be applied easily elsewhere, this is not the place to look. It is one attempt to record changes which otherwise become lost over time as approaches which were once thought to be innovative become an accepted way of working. This chapter looks at the context of mental health care in the city of Manchester, the response to the White Paper changes, management reforms and working with other agencies.

The city of Manchester of the early 1990s mirrors many of the contradictions and opportunities of Britain as a whole. The city illustrates the movement away from a local economy based on the old manufacturing industries towards the growth of a service economy. This change has brought a wealth to the city through the growth of financial institutions and the service sector ranging from leisure and the arts to high technology support services. The city is a partner in one of the fastest growing airports in the world and has made bids to stage the Olympic games. By the late 1980s over two-thirds of all employment was in the services and increasingly those new jobs which were created were in relatively poorly paid parts of the economy such as the food industry. In the years between 1961 and 1983 one in eight manufacturing jobs in the city were lost, some 160 000 jobs.

Throughout the 1980s Manchester City Council (1986, 1988, 1989) carried out three major studies of social change and poverty in the city. In the last of these, Manchester City Council (1989) produced evidence which suggested that of the total population of 450 000, some 30 000 lived in homes without essential heating and 20 000 homes were affected by damp. One in three citizens lived in poverty in that they lacked three or more necessities; one in six people lacked five or more necessities; one in ten lacked seven or more necessities. The factors which influenced this position are perhaps predictable, as they include high correlations between unemployment, single parent families, disability and old age. The survey carried out by the City Council clearly linked the existence of poverty to dependence on the social security system as one-third of the sample contained households with at least one person receiving social security benefits. Between one-third and one-half of those households surveyed which contained persons with a disability were classified as being in poverty. The report of the survey concluded that deprivation in Manchester was widespread and nearly one-third of households surveyed were found to go without three or more household or personal items, and were therefore regarded as living in poverty. Of these people, there were almost one in ten who could be classified as intensely deprived.

Health and poverty are linked in both obvious and subtle ways, as was demonstrated by the report of the Manchester joint Consultative Committee (1986). This study by the Community Physicians of the three Manchester District Health

Authorities and the City Planning Department highlighted the growth of inequalities in health within an overall context of improvements in health. Evidence is produced to show that in Manchester child deaths have reduced dramatically throughout the twentieth century. In 1901 40% of all deaths in the city were of children under 5 years, by 1981 this had fallen to 1.2%. However Manchester residents had a higher proportion of premature deaths for those aged under 65 when compared to the population as a whole. At the other end of the age spectrum, almost one child in ten born in Manchester was likely to have a recorded low weight at birth which is a third higher than the national average. The Report also makes clear that within the city there are marked inequalities of health between differing neighbourhoods and wards. The population of the inner city covered by Central Manchester Health Authority had some of the highest indicators of ill health. This population experienced a higher death rate than the national average; some 80% higher for those under the age of 65. For specific causes of death the rate was even higher; death from lung cancer was over twice the national average, as were respiratory diseases. In contrast, the figures for the more prosperous wards of south Manchester showed a lower than average death rate for the under 65s compared to the national average. So whilst Manchester as a whole had significant levels of poverty and there was a well-researched relationship between poverty and ill-health; within Manchester itself there were significant inequalities with the most deprived part of the inner city being the poorest materially, and health-wise.

## HEALTH AND POVERTY: AN ENDURING RELATIONSHIP

The inner city areas of Manchester are largely those areas covered by the Central Manchester Health Authority; the area is divided into nine electoral ward boundaries and neighbourhoods. The area is compact – little more than 12 square miles in area with a resident population of approximately 122 000 people. The inner city is an island of poverty within the commercial centre of one of the country's major commercial cities. In contrast to the growing service sector of the city, especially the financial services sector the nine wards present a picture of inner city blight, urban decay and poverty.

The story of central Manchester is the stereotypical case of the inner city in decline. The resident population is reducing year by year but the level of need is increasing, as reflected by the demand for health and welfare services. Whilst it is estimated that the total number of residents will fall throughout the 1990s there is evidence from the Office of Population, Census and Statistics (OPCS 1986, 1990) that the numbers of people under 5 and over 75 will increase. These are two of the most vulnerable and dependent groups in the population and they offer a particular challenge for health and social services.

Central Manchester Health Authority (1989) reviewed the data on the characteristics of the local population and the impact of poverty on the health of residents of the inner city. One of the marked features of the population was that more than one person in six was born outside the United Kingdom with the largest groups being the Irish, Afro-Caribbeans and people from Pakistan. The Authority estimated that in three of the nine wards over 20% of the population lived in a household headed by a person born in the New Common-wealth or Pakistan. These wards were Longsight, Hulme and Moss Side. The Report makes powerful links between life in the inner city and the growth of poverty. It is argued that over the last two decades, for example, the level of unemployment has increased from 10 to 36%. Other independent comment-ators have also singled out parts of central Manchester as being socially deprived. The British Medical Association (1987) cited the findings of the Jarman index of factors which indicate social deprivation. This work looked at all 192 District Health authorities in England and Wales and clustered the scores within the 14 Regional Health Authorities. The conclusions are stark. The evidence of the Jarman index of eight factors of deprivation showed that Tower Hamlets in East London was the single most deprived health area in Britain; the second and third most deprived areas in the index were Hulme and Moss Side in central Manchester. The research carried out by the Central Manchester Health Authority and published in 1989 looked to the use of standardized mortality ratios (SMRs) as a way of statistically representing the ill health of the local population. This technique corrects the differences in age structure and represents the number of expected deaths overall as 100. The report commented that for Ardwick,

Moss Side and Hulme the SMR was 178; this means that, on average, residents are 78% more likely to die than in the country as a whole.

As part of the preparation for the introduction of the *Caring for People* initiative the multi-agency Joint Planning Group for Mental Health produced a report on the shortfall in services for care in the community in central Manchester. This Central Manchester JPTMH (1990) examined the implications of the changes for the statutory and voluntary organizations in the area. As part of the evidence gathered by the group there was a particular interest shown in the services for people with long-term mental illnesses as they featured as a group of core users of mental health services. The data showed that the health service in central Manchester provided services for 422 people in this group of which 102 received specialist community support; 25 were in-patients, 275 were provided for by Community Psychiatric Nurses in the community and 20 attended the Psychiatric Day Hospital. A further 330 people received specialist mental health services from the two social services offices and 60 had a service from the local authority community network. This meant that over 800 central area residents received a service either from the health service or from social services. It proved impossible to gather reliable data to reflect the mental health work of the local voluntary sector. The report concluded that a spectrum of care was required to meet the needs of the resident population, especially the long-term mentally ill. The settings suggested for care included domiciliary support to people in their own homes; day and respite care, sheltered housing residential care and long-term hospital care. The report also highlighted the fact that there are people in receipt of services which are inappropriate for their needs and reference was made to a 1986 survey which identified 174 people in such circumstances. The report highlighted the lack of reliable epidemiological data to make proper assessments of the needs of the local population as a whole. The report also questioned the usefulness of the distinction between 'social' need and 'health' needs of the chronically mentally ill. *What was needed, it was argued, was not a way of distinguishing between the responsibilities of health and the social services agencies, but greater integration of services.*

Almost 150 years ago, Engels, in his study of social life and wealth, commented on the work of the Manchester Royal Infirmary in providing medical services to the poor of the first industrial city in the world. The Royal Infirmary continues to provide services to people in inner city Manchester albeit from a new site developed before the First World War. The point has been made already that there are a number of independent sources of evidence which establish central Manchester as a major island of poverty in a prosperous region. As a consequence of this deprivation the health needs of the population are significantly greater in both magnitude and severity when compared to other, similarly-sized populations. The next part of this chapter will examine the way in which mental health services have been organized to respond to the mental health needs of the inner city population as well as other users of services.

## PROVIDING SERVICES IN CENTRAL MANCHESTER: A CASE STUDY

As a result of the changes introduced following *Working for Patients* discussed in Chapter 5, Central Manchester health providers became part of the first wave of self-governing trusts in April 1991. In many parts of the country the first trusts were often single units or hospitals and this was in contrast to the approach taken by those in central Manchester. With the separation of the purchasing function from the provider role the Central Manchester Health Authority became the purchaser of most health services for local residents. All of the providers in the pre-1991 health authority, including the Manchester Royal Infirmary, St Mary's Hospital, the Royal Eye Hospital, the Dental Hospital and all Community Services, became part of an integrated new trust. The task of the new 'Manchester Central Hospitals and Community Care NHS Trust' was to provide services to the local resident population and to people from other health authorities, as agreed by specific contracts for services. The largest single contract was with the Central Manchester Health Authority to provide a range of hospital and community services to the residents of the nine wards of central Manchester. In addition to the role of direct provider of services, the Trust also undertook to continue a long-standing commitment to teaching and research, especially through medical education provided by the University of Manchester.

Health service organization and management can be seen as being unrelated to the real business of delivering care to individuals. It will be argued here that such a view leads to a very partial understanding of the issues involved in providing mental health services. To explore the connections between the management of resources and the provision of patient care, this chapter will look at the experience of mental health services in central Manchester as a case study of change. This will focus on two particular issues: first, the local implications of wider changes in the NHS and, second, the local experience of one area working to provide mental health services.

Like many of the older teaching hospitals those of the Central Manchester Trust are situated in the inner city and are surrounded by some of the most deprived neighbourhoods in the country. Much of the central part of the area is given over to property owned and run by institutions such as the University, Polytechnic and the NHS. Surrounding these institutions are the nine ward neighbourhoods which comprise the local resident population. The area is cut through with major roads leading to and from the commercial centre of the city. During their construction much of the old terraced housing was demolished to make way for high rise housing on large estates. The most notable of these in the central area are Hulme and Moss Side where the substandard terraces of the Victorian period were replaced in the 1960s by municipal housing which has proved to be both less durable and less socially cohesive than the homes it replaced. In such a setting the Department of Psychiatry provides a range of services for local residents and for people referred from outside the immediate area. This chapter will look at the issues facing practitioners and managers alike in managing these services in a period of radical change.

MENTAL HEALTH AND MENTAL ILLNESS SERVICES

The Department of Psychiatry is relatively young as it has existed in its present form since the beginning of the 1980s. It is an integral part of the Manchester Central Trust (the provider) and as such it is required to negotiate, manage and provide a range of services required by the Central Manchester Health Authority (the purchaser) as well as provide services to other purchasers within the North West Region and from other Districts. The Department has three major functions:

1.  To provide **patient care** by developing a comprehensive range of services for residents of central Manchester as well as specialist referrals from other areas.
2.  To **teach** medical, nursing, occupational therapy, psychology and social work undergraduates and post-graduates.
3.  To carry out **research** as agreed within the Department and with external funders.

To organize and manage these three key objectives as part of a developing service requires some agreement on the values which inform practice and policy-making. These values are the produce of custom and practice as well as the produce of a concerted attempt to clarify the beliefs which underpin thinking within the Department. What follows is a description of the a new way of managing mental health services in central Manchester through the establishment of a clinical directorate. Before discussing the way in which the directorate was established and the formal organizational structure, it is useful to set out some of the key ideas adopted within the Department. The last decade has seen the emergence of a service which has a commitment to an integrated model of care which includes both hospital and community services; one is interdependent upon the other. This was important for the overall development of the department and the directorate in that a range of services were to be managed from within the one organization. In addition, there was a well-established tradition of working in partnership with a range of agencies, especially in the non-statutory sector already working in the local neighbourhood. This is an important point as it is well recognized that health provision is only part of the picture when the mental health needs of a community is considered. There are many agencies who contribute overall to the provision of mental health services, especially where the health side is only partly developed.

As with all parts of the NHS after April 1991, services within the central area are increasingly focused on the need to meet contracts agreed with purchasers. These contracts will eventually specify the quality, cost and volume of services provided for each area of speciality. In the initial period of the contractual relationship the task is to continue to provide the level of service as before. This 'block contract' arrangement may be varied in future years through negotiation between the purchasers and the providers. It is also likely that the overall numbers of purchasers may increase with the new responsibilities of the Family Health Service Authority and the appearance of GP fund-holding practices. The three principles referred to above: integrated care between hospital and community, partnership with local agencies and the rise of a contract culture played a significant part in the thinking about the type of management which was necessary for the future of mental health services in central Manchester.

The approaches developed and applied in the department are drawn from a rich variety of sources, some of which are home grown and others are taken from agencies in other places trying to tackle similar problems. What became clear is that the mechanical application of ideas and approaches grafted on from outside and separate from the daily life of the department would not work as an imposed solution. It was those ideas which could be adapted for the local situation which proved to be the most valuable and durable.

It is one thing to subscribe to a set of principles which can be set down in a document, but it is quite another to try to develop this into a series of aims which every member of the Department can own as their own. Therefore, as well as the general principles outlined above there has been an attempt made to set out the aims of the service in a way which informs everyday practice as well as overall policy. Following consultation with the professional staff within the Department it was agreed that the single overall aim of the Department was to provide the best possible standard of assessment and treatment for people with psychiatric disorders and disabilities. The approach to be used being one which sought to integrate physical, psychological, social, cultural and ethnic aspects of patient care. In short the task is to provide quality services which are complete and appropriate. Achieving this laudable objective involved the promotion of high standards of training and staff development for professionals of all disciplines and developing the approach into a practical process.

As a result of the discussions set out above which took place over a period of a year, six key aims were agreed which stated that all services should be:

1. personal;
2. multidisciplinary;
3. local;
4. continuing;
5. specialist;
6. efficient.

If these approaches are to be more than rhetorical they need to be expressed in greater detail and spelt out for both service-users and providers.

To claim that a service is *personal* means that treatment has to be based on the specific needs of the individual patient or service-user; therefore their rights and wishes have to be respected at all times. Whenever possible individuals and their carers should be involved in a participative way in planning and treatment programmes. The idea that services should be *multi-disciplinary* is partly a recognition of some current practice but also a statement about the need to change as other skills are developed. In order to provide a comprehensive service there is a need to have access to a range of skills and disciplines including the teaching function both inside and outside the Department. One of the key aims is to provide a *local* service especially to offer treatment in patients' own homes whenever possible. For some patients in-patient and day-patient care will be necessary when it is inappropriate to provide services in a community setting. However, as with central government policy, the aim overall is to provide more services in the community, especially through closer work with the local authority and the independent sector. There is much to be done to promote closer links with family members and informal carers, especially in providing support for them to continue to care. The continued development of innovative local projects to treat and support patients in the community is one key feature of this strategy. There is a practical difficulty with this aim in a teaching setting, in that a significant number of service-users referred to the Department come from areas other than central Manchester. One of the tasks facing the Department is to find ways of ensuring that appropriate community services are available to these people. The aim of providing a *continuing* service to patients follows on from the last comment in that it is essential to the service that there is continuity of care across hospital and community settings. In particular, the long-term mentally ill are being encouraged to live as independently as possible through opportunities in day care, vocational work, leisure and recreational facilites, as well as supported residential care. One of the key aims of the Department is to further develop *specialist* services as part of the range of facilities offered and to ensure that the management of the Department reflects the organization of services. Lastly, the Department aims to offer an *efficient* service which makes optimum use of the financial, staffing and material resources available as well as monitoring and evaluating the standards of care provided.

Part of the process of change was to develop a good working relationship with the independent sector. This was achieved with four local agencies: the Afro-Caribbean Mental Health Group; the Zion Resource Centre in Hulme; Manchester Housing Consortium for Mental Health; and the Psychiatric Social Work Education Centre. These organizations made available fresh voices and ideas to facilitate change within the health service, and mental health services in particular.

MANAGING CHANGE IN A CONTRACT CULTURE

It has already been explained that services provided by the department of Psychiatry and the Trust overall are regulated and negotiated through the use of contracts which introduced the first steps in the development of the internal market within the NHS. Clearly in order to enter into a contract process it is essential that services can be described and managed in a way which is both understandable and acceptable to the purchaser of services. These rather cold business and legalistic terms mask a richer and more complex process which will take several years for the NHS as a whole to resolve. However, to understand the application in one Department requires further explanation and enquiry. In order to work as a successful part of the Trust the Department of Psychiatry has to organize its activities in a way which could ensure that it met the range of contractual obligations. This objective gives rise to three major questions:

1.  How are services organized?
2.  What is the management structure?
3.  What is the management process?

## Organization of services

The Department of Psychiatry is comprised of over 400 people from a range of disciplines working on 11 separate sites and incurring costs of over $5 million at 1992/93 prices. The work of the Department is divided into six major areas of patient care which forms the basic core organization for clinical work:

1.  Child and Adolescent Services
2.  General Adult Psychiatry
3.  Regional Speciality in Psychotherapy
4.  Community Drugs Team
5.  Rehabilitation
6.  Psychiatry of Old Age

The management structure of the Department changed radically with the introduction of the changes in health and community care provision. To be precise the changes were introduced in order to position the department to deliver quality services within the contractual framework. Prior to the development of the self-governing Trust, the department of Psychiatry was part of a community unit of management which included a collection of disparate services under an administrative and managerial umbrella. There was a marked separation between the clinical activity of the Department and the financial control and management function. The idea of service planning, development and change in essence rested on the quality of the relationships between the individuals involved rather than as an organic and natural part of the management process. The distinction between clinical and managerial issues was relatively arbitrary and the priorities of the Department tended to be set in response to in-year budget pressures rather than by an agreed business plan for each speciality driven by clinical and user needs. The specialist areas of service did exist, but they had an internal life of their own which was divorced from the management structure and process. The problem facing the Department was to find a way to link the agendas for clinical services with the need to manage a service in a changing political, financial and professional climate.

In addition to the weak links between people providing patient care and the management control function, there were a number of other issues which tended to cut across the management of the Department such as the interests of differing professional disciplines. There were specialist services but they did not have identifiable budgets of their own; there were separate disciplines which worked together but were not responsible through a coherent line management structure within that service. Some of the services operated on a number of sites with little interplay between them or even any real appreciation of the relative value of the work of other practitioners. The task for the department as a whole was to find a management structure which was appropriate for the range of activities provided and which strengthened the ability of the Department to survive, develop and prosper under the changes being introduced. In short, how could the Department find an alternative management structure to ensure that there was a direct relationship between patient activity and management decision-making?

Over a period of a year prior to the introduction of the health changes and the emergence of the Trust the Department invested a considerable amount of time and energy in looking critically at the existing organization. This included a series of meetings with key stake holders from a range of disciplines and services in order to establish the appetite for change. From this there merged a statement of four key management objectives:

1. To provide a clear line of management responsibility directly from the Chief Executive of the Trust through to each area of specialist patient care.
2. To set out clear objectives for performance accountability for each specialist area of service.
3. To ensure that the department is successful in providing agreed quality and volumes of care within the resources available.

4. To enable professional staff to become stake-holders in specialist services by shaping future services.

These four objectives, which addressed the core issues of responsibility, accountability, resource management and ownership, formed the basis of the discussion of the management structure which was to emerge for the Department. The subsequent discussion and debate lead to a demand to increase the degree of local control exercised by managers in the Department and in turn this lead to the call for the creation of a separate psychiatry grouping as an alternative to the existing community unit of management. This new grouping was the Clinical Directorate of Psychiatry which was created to ensure that appropriate mental health services could be provided through contracts within the self-governing trust. There were two key reasons for the creation of this new form of organization: first, to establish a direct line management relationship to the Trust and, second, to develop devolved decision-making in the Department of Psychiatry. This new body emphasized specialist services as the core elements of the Directorate and therefore the six areas of speciality formed the cornerstone of the directorate.

## Management structure

The structure of the Clinical Directorate of Psychiatry developed out of the experience of delivering services and through the use of the Resource Management Initiative (RMI) established by the NHS. This focused attention on the core relationship between management and clinical services which involved a better understanding of the financial and resource consequences of clinical decision-making. The resource management initiative within the NHS provided an opportunity to recognize the key relationship which was that in order to achieve good quality, effective patient care, it was necessary to involve professionals in management. The structure which was created is illustrated in Figure 8.1. The Executive group consisted of the Clinical Director, Director of Nursing and Quality Assurance, Medical representative and the General Manager. These arrangements were discussed with the Chief Executive of the Trust and given his approval. In all within

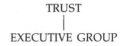

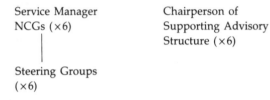

MANAGEMENT BOARD

Service Manager
NCGs (×6)

Steering Groups
(×6)

Directorate Working Groups
e.g. Health and Safety
    Division of Medicine
    Audit

**Figure 8.1** Clinical directorate: simplified structure.

the Trust there were likely to be some 15 separate Directorates. These would relate to the Chief Executive and the Trust Board through a new Assistant Chief Executive who would be primarily concerned with the business performance of each Directorate rather than care policy or operational matters. There would also be a new forum for Clinical Directors across the Trust to meet together and advise the Chief Executive on clinical concerns and the development of policies and practices of the trust.

## Management process

One of the tasks of managers is to live within the resources available but also maximize the use of those resources. Equally important, however, is the task of producing evidence of need for the service, and advising those providers who allocate resources or negotiate with the purchasers of the gap between current services and the needs identified. Thus, the elements of the management process include the following:

1. To establish a dialogue with professional staff and service-users to ensure that the experience of providing and receiving services is reflected in management decision-making.
2. To enable direct service-providers to relate their professional practice to the wider issues of social policy and the political climate.
3. To provide evidence rather than anecdote to support arguments for change.
4. To work with others in the Department to establish an atmosphere which is both supportive and challenging.
5. To take responsibility for issues which would prove to be difficult or unacceptable for any one discipline or professional.
6. To work with other professionals to help them to do their job to the best effect.

To initiate this process and produce tangible benefits for psychiatric services the Directorate looked at some of the obstacles to the management process. Three key ideas emerged from these discussions. First, there was a marked absence of reliable financial information and as a result it was impossible to produce accurate costs for services delivered. Second, decision-making was concentrated in senior managers' hands to such a degree that many decisions were taken at some distance from the delivery of direct patient care. Third, there was a need to involve middle management staff in the process of developing new approaches to care and management through a staff development.

The directorate Management Board which consisted of the Executive Group (4), Service Managers (6) and representatives from the Support Structure (5). The formal relationship between the Management Board and the Executive is advisory on matters of policy and practice within the Directorate. The Service Manager works closely with a designated medical consultant to advise and negotiate contracts between the Trust and the District health Authority purchaser. The steering Groups are convened by the Service Managers and they will reflect the range of disciplines involved in a particular service although this could be augmented by representatives from other agencies if desired. The task of the Steering Group is to produce three papers each year including a prospectus of services provided; a review of operational policies including quality and audit processes being used, and a service and business plan showing current costs, in year changes and proposals for change.

A key part of the management process within the Clinical Directorate of Psychiatry is the ability of managers and professional staff to match information on clinical activity to other indicators on performance. To help in this process three key sources of data were identified. First, the Department of Health Korner system, which proved to be a poor tool to account for community services. Second, the Psychiatric Case Register (PCR) which captures data on all medical consultations and attempts to establish a longitudinal record of patient care. Third, the Patient Administration System (PAS) which is the key data source for all patient contacts across the Trust and which plays an important part in the data used for contracts and income. It became clear that there was a pressing need for the PCR and PAS systems will be linked together as a significant part of the demographic information is common between them and therefore involves a degree of duplication of effort. The use of information systems will be discussed further in Chapter 10 as there are unresolved ethical and managerial problems, especially in the establishment of case registers.

This chapter is unlike others in this book in that it is an account of a process which is undergoing continual change. The changes referred to above are the practical implications of the wider changes set out in the government white papers discussed in Chapters 4 and 5. It is important to try to capture the immediacy of these changes and the discussions which surround them as it is almost impossible to reconstruct it from the official papers at a later date. The discussion on management above contains one essential truth which is that better patient care is achieved when clinical professionals, be they doctors, nurses or occupational therapists, work together with managers to achieve common goals. The actual structure which emerges from these discussions is almost necessarily a temporary arrangement, although it may last for several years.

Management itself is a pragmatic process; a way of coping with the uncertainty of a changing external world of politics, funding and expectations and an internal world of professional ambitions and developing skills.

## PERSPECTIVES

The demand for health care in the widest sense is unstable as the boundaries are moved on from generation to generation. The evidence referred to above attempts to make the case that areas such as Central Manchester make greater demands on mental health services than other areas of the country. In the mental health field the NHS is only one of a number of agencies with responsibilities. The departments of the local authority such as social services and housing as well as the central government-managed social security system also deal with people with mental illness. Some of these services are available to residents as a right, although much of the anecdotal accounts by service-users gives testimony to the fragmented and un-coordinated way that services are deployed.

In response to the problem of fragmented services it was hoped in the late 1970s that a new form of joint planning would result in better services for people with mental illness. There is no evidence that joint planning has worked in the mental health field in Manchester as much of the time is spent discussing the use of joint finance rather than joint planning. What was intended to be marginal money to facilitate innovation has become an end in itself. This is perhaps indicative of the parlous state of funding for mental health in general. In Manchester the city council Social Services Department has experienced sustained cuts in the annual budget since the late 1980s. Paradoxically these cuts have been implemented in the same period as the introduction of the care in the community initiative which brought with it a range of new responsibilities. There is nothing new in the fact that that circumstances arise in which greater demands are made on an already over-burdened system at the very time when the means to provide existing services is being eroded. Mental health care in Manchester as in many places is being provided in in circumstances which are not of the providers or users choosing.

Difficult decisions have to be made on priorities, the use of resources and the development of services; in other words the management of care.

Chapter 9 will look at a set of issues which are rather wider than the local experience of one inner city area responding to the changing climate of health and social care. These are some of the central and unresolved issues which confront mental health services and those who use them in the last part of the twentieth century.

# From here to alternatives

## THE COST AND QUALITY PROBLEM

Much of the history of mental health policy and practice has been concerned with the relationship between cost and quality although this has often been veiled in other terms such as resources and un-met needs. This chapter looks at three issues in the development of mental health services: the economic cost of mental health problems, the place of quality of life issues in mental health services and an alternative process to help clarify decision-making for professionals and users alike.

The problem of fragmented services for the mentally ill pre-dates the 1990s reforms of the NHS and the changes in the provision of community services. There has been a growing recognition in government thinking of the impact of mental illness on both individuals and society as a whole; examples of this were cited in the earlier discussion on the White Papers of the 1970s. However, this recognition has translated itself into an uneven set of arrangements for the care of the mentally ill with significant sums of money being used in un-coordinated ways.

One of the features of the problems of funding mental health care is the emergence of unlikely alliances of groups who super-ficially have little in common. The lure of care in the community and the move away from hospital-based services has been applauded by political thinkers of both left and right. To the left the move towards community provision is an expression of personal liberation and a shift from institutionalized care. To the political right the development of community care is seen as a way of reducing costs and expenditure through hospital closures. However, the change may highlight an undercurrent of change which, in the longer run, has a more profound effect on the way services are perceived and delivered.

The Mental Health Foundation (1990) produced evidence to show that 6 million people in Britain suffer from some form of mental illness each year. This means that 1:10 of the population is estimated at some point in their lifetime to be in need of professional mental health services. These figures are based on the clinical coding of general practitioners consultations using a standardized format. This means that mental illness is three times more common than cancer and 3200 times more common than AIDS. Of these 6 million people some 3.7 million were classified as having a severe mental illness. This figure is contrasted with the 58 000 people in mental hospitals at any one time. For most people in contact with specialist mental health services, care is provided in the community through day hospital, out-patient, community clinic, community nurses or other forms of intervention. However the hospital is doggedly persistent as the focus of attention for mental health services.

The Department of Social Security (1989) estimated that between the NHS, Local authorities and social security departments over £3 billion is spent each year in providing for the mentally ill. If the estimated cost of lost days of work are added to this figure using the research of the Office of Population Census and Statistics (OPCS) (1988) then £3.7 billion needs to be added to the total. This means that best estimates indicate that the financial cost of mental illness in Britain from direct costs of services and from lost working days totals £6.8 billion per annum.

In looking at the way the money and resources are spent on the direct provision of services a number of questions are raised about the priorities in mental health care. The government Central Statistics Office (CSO) reported in 1990 that the cost of in-patient services accounted for 71% of the cost of direct NHS care for the mentally ill. This is despite in-patient care accounting for less than 60 000 of the population in need of specialist psychiatric services. In a study of the relative costs of hospital versus community care Knapp *et al.* (1990) looked at the costs of providing for people who had previously been long-stay hospital residents. Knapp is at pains to highlight some of the qualifications involved in this type of research as he emphasizes the needs for costs to be comprehensive: to include wide variations; to make comparisons cautiously; and to work towards relating costing data to outcomes for the patient. Knapp concluded this piece of research with the comment that community care costs are lower than hospital care costs for the full populations of the two hospitals undergoing closure. He emphasizes, however, the need to distinguish between the support required for this group of ex-patients and the community care costs of providing for the acutely mentally ill in the community. A similar point applies to the earlier discussion on Warner (1985) and Beecham *et al.* (1991) and the decline of the mental hospital population. Those people who have endured long-stays in the old hospitals and those people who are chronically mentally ill in the community may have very differing characteristics and needs.

The resource problem faced by mental health services is threefold:

1. The level of funding to provide for the mentally ill is not only inadequate for the scale of need, but the resources are fragmented between differing agencies of central and local government.
2. The greater part of the resources within the health service are tied up in the hospital in-patient service where a small minority of patients are treated, whilst the great majority in community services receive the smallest allocation of resources.
3. The fragmentation which is evident in direct patient care between health and social care is mirrored in the way in which resources are allocated and managed.

Resources for mental health services are not provided or planned on a coherent or rational basis as they are in competition for scarce resources from other services provided by the respective organizations. Within the health service the acute hospital service dominates thinking and expenditure whereas in the social services child care still receives the lion's share of the available resources. This point is not to decry the importance of hospital or child care services, but to highlight the distance which exists between the rhetoric of care in the community and the practice of setting priorities for expenditure.

## FUNDING FRAGMENTED SERVICES

For the last 40 years and more health and social services have been organized and provided to respond to the *demand for services* rather than the *needs of individuals or communities*. This point may seem petty and esoteric but it goes right to the heart of the dilemmas facing those who have to plan and provide services. The demand for services is a reflection of what is currently provided, limited by resources or imagination, whereas the need for services is a direct and personal expression of the support required by individuals. Goldberg and Huxley (1980) make the point that what a given society understands by psychiatric illness is defined by the characteristics of the referral pathway to the psychiatrist. If alternative pathways can be found and new services developed in response to this, then the understanding of mental illness changes. If the Goldberg and Huxley idea is developed further then some of the inherent weaknesses of recent approaches to community care begin to appear. The strength of hospital-based systems of care is that they have a single institutional base from which to operate. This can lead to cohesion amongst the staff group and a degree of negotiating power as regards funding and resources. For services provided in the community there is no such institutional base and much of the cohesion which can exist is either a function of the personal relations of those working together or a shared set of values in community provision.

Curiously, both the hospital and the community form of provision share a central weakness in that they tend to have a single means of entry to the service; hospitals may be criticized for being too restrictive and controlling for the patient and community services too ill-defined with their client group for specific conditions to be treated. Hudson (1989) makes the point that one of the problems of collaboration between health and social services agencies is the implied threat to the autonomy of the other agency. It is argued that acquiring the resources of another agency is not a good basis for future partnership between organizations.

In the world of separated purchasers and providers, within both the health and social services organizations, the setting of priorities will be the responsibility of the purchasers. They are the people who will have to decide between competing priorities for services funded through cash-limited budgets. In the mental health field the purchaser of services has to make strategic choices which establish a balance between three competing axis; acute versus chronic needs, hospital versus community provision and public versus private services.

The balance between acute and chronic services should be a direct function of the population served; in areas under heavy pressure such as the inner city there may be inadequate resources to meet either of these needs. The dichotomy of hospital versus community provision will reflect the values of the organization, as well as the ability to meet complex needs in the community. The choice between public as opposed to private provision is increasingly a daily dilemma for those managing the care of the elderly as the standards of the local authority residential home may not be able to match that of the private home inspected by the same local authority. In all of these dilemmas there are a range of judgements to be made regarding the preferences of the individual patient, local experience of services, budget pressures and the status of mental health services overall. Each issue presents problems of cost and quality which have to be confronted in the negotiation of service contracts. It is not sufficient to assume that the person in hospital receives more personal care or the community alternative is cheaper. Such assumptions are only of use as rhetorical debating points; each locality and those involved as service-users, providers and purchasers must find their own way to resolve these complex and interrelated problems. The emergence of comprehensive and appropriate mental health services can not be imposed as a single blueprint from outside or from above. But such comprehensive services must be developed in each locality in order to ensure that the range and quality of services available and the services available to local residents are not a function of where they live.

The movement towards community-based services did not arise out of a single event or belief as it is a complex blend of economics, patient preference and the inability to maintain the old hospital system. What is clear is that patients and referrers who look for mental health services seek a range of help. There is a place for the hospital as well as the community as part of the comprehensive range of care. The problem is to find an approach which helps to establish a balance and relationship between hospital and community-based services. The answer to this most persistent and complex of problems is being tackled in a variety of novel ways. The climate of change in the NHS from the late 1980s led to a greater concentration on the outcomes produced by services rather than the traditional output measures (see Creed *et al.*, 1990, and Dean and Gadd, 1990). One of the ways in which this has been approached over the last decade has been through the use of quality measures to try to establish the impact of services on the individuals who use them.

Much of the health and social work literature refers to 'quality' as if it were a single thing which everybody understood in the same way. In fact, the emergence of quality as an issue in health care and the personal social services is a product of the 1980s and it appeared out of the commercial and industrial world. Much has been written about the role of quality; the total quality organization, quality standards and quality assurance. The contracts agreed by the purchasing health authorities and the provider units talk of quality as part of the three cornerstones of the service contract; the other two are patient volumes and cost. Quality as a concept has become a new watchword in health care and as such it is prone to be used in a random and imprecise way. It is often used as a weapon with which to win an argument, in that everyone is required to subscribe to quality; although what is often meant is high quality provision at lower cost. Attempts to clarify the concept include Bigelow *et al.* (1982) and Lehman, Possidente and Hawker (1986) who studied a group of chronically mentally ill patients living in the community and concluded that residents' perception of living conditions was more favourable in the community than in hospital. The residents had more disposable income and they felt that they were less likely to be subject to assault than when in hospital. Lehman *et al.* (1986) explained the differences in patients' perception of their living conditions as a function of their sense of well-being. The study concluded that if the old hospitals must be *retained*, then they ought to be *maintained* as well. In an earlier study Lehman

(1983) looked at the notion of well-being as part of a quality of life measure in a survey of mental health service-users in Los Angeles board and care homes. Lehman used three measures in the study; an account of personal characteristics, objective circumstances and subjective indicators to construct a measure of global well-being. Lehman concluded that this measure had five characteristics which included personal safety; social relations, finances, leisure time and health care. He further developed this approach in the Lehman *et al.* (1988) survey which compared hospital and community care experiences and outcomes.

Oliver (1991) gives an account of the application of a quality of life measure developed from the original research by Lehman referred to above. Oliver concludes with three points: first, quality of life assessments can put individual assessment at the centre of service planning. Second, the outcomes of human services are to do with their clients' life conditions. Third, health and social services authorities typically employ different information in planning their services. These seemingly simple statements say something profound about the way in which health and social care agencies regard their users. The approach being developed by Oliver is rooted in the joint experience of the service provider and the service-user and with application and a commitment to researching practice quality of of life measures can be an invaluable tool.

The idea of a high quality service which is capable of overcoming the old dichotomies between health and social care and hospital and the community is enormously attractive to those who seek an integrated and comprehensive range of services. This has been recognized by some of those involved in drafting the 1990s reforms of community provision and searching for a planning system which allows innovative services to be developed. The Social Services Inspectorate (1990) argued for the need for effective machinery to prevent individuals becoming the causalties of unresolved boundary disputes between agencies. Kingsley and Towell (1989) looked at the issues involved in designing local processes for the development of mental health services. They criticized the traditional approach to centralized planning which emphasized 'top down' planning as a way of frustrating local innovation and unnecesssarily restricting the emergence of good ideas for the development of local services. What they did not mention was the state of joint planning between local authorities, the health service and the voluntary sector. This has been organized through a hierarchy of committees from client specific Planning Teams, Joint Care Planning Teams and Joint Consultative Committees at the apex of the system. Sadly, much of the work of these groups has focused on the joint finance monies rather than on strategic joint planning. Joint finance was never more than marginal money to act as 'pump priming' to change in the larger system. Increasingly through the 1980s joint finance consistantly became the topic of planning teams discussion, rather than the core task of jointly planning and coordinating services and developments.

The experience of joint planning, collaboration and attempts at organizational restructuring have failed to deal with some of the fundamental problems of mental health needs. Much of the planning has been imposed from above without access to the daily experience of providing mental health care or from being a service-user. Up to the beginning of the 1990s this situation was allowed to continue as the consequences were limited to those in the mental health field. Mental health services were but one small voice amongst many. For both health and social services the consequences of failing to develop joint plans and strategies were limited. However with White Paper policies that separated the purchaser and provider functions the situation changed. The White Papers reflected a change in official thinking which looked to a market economy approach to health and social care. The service-user could be seen as a consumer which in turn implied that the user had not only rights, but choices. The task of drafting of the community care plan fell to social services, who were obliged to consult and agree with other statutory agencies including community (user) representatives.

The second part of this chapter will explore some of the possibilities for change in the management of policy and practice and present an alternative strategy for mental health professionals and service-users alike.

## TOWARDS AN ALTERNATIVE STRATEGY

The alternative approach put forward here is *not* a model of care, but rather a process for joint decision-making. It is intended to be non-prescriptive in terms of the professional judgements involved or the form of assessment and treatment offered. It concentrates on the way in which decisions are taken and seeks to establish a process which allows a range of voices to be heard whilst coordinating the efforts of individuals and services to meet jointly agreed aims. Central to this approach is the acceptance of the idea that the service-user must be actively involved in the process if it is to be successful.

The White Papers discussed in Chapters 4 and 5 comment on the role of the service-user in the mental health care system as 'patient' and 'client'. The White Papers suggest that the user is likely to find a new role centre stage in the reformed health and social care system, especially in a system which explicitly emphasizes consumer choice and where the money follows the patient. What is more likely to happen if current customs and practice remain in place is that the service-user will be represented by proxy, whether by the general practitioner, Community Health Council or the purchaser. The problem is especially acute for those people who are being treated in the mental health system. So often one of the consequences of mental illness is either the onset of a sense of personal powerlessness or an expectation in society that the person is unable to voice a coherent opinion. Therefore, any strategy for mental health services has to meet a number of differing needs simultaneously, in particular the needs of a range of different interests. Jowell (1991) looked at the possibility of there being shared values within a mental health service and she highlighted a number of key points in the process. Jowell considered seven factors to be of particular importance including consultation, self-determination, individually appropriate support, the use of the least restrictive setting, minimum segregation, accessability and culturally appropriate support. These points are laudable enough but they will only mean something if they can be translated into a working plan to deliver individual care and monitor service performance in a way that is satisfactory to service-users, professionals and the purchaser.

The clues to achieving this objective are all around us, rooted in the experience of delivering care and in the judgements made by users and professionals alike. The 1990s reforms of health and social care provide an opportunity to reformulate some of these ideas into a novel solution to the old problem of how can different organizations work together to the benefit of the service-user. In particular, the central question which needs to be addressed is how can services be organized and delivered in such a way that they are no longer fragmented? There are essentially two alternative answers to this problem: firstly, to establish a new **structure** whereby a single agency has responsibility for all aspects of mental health services. Secondly, to find a **process** which allows the agencies to work in a partnerhsip which emphasizes the process rather than the structure. The first of these solutions is one which has been demonstrated in America and is the subject of part of Chapter 7. In the political climate of the early 1990s, with the degree of uncertainty which informs local government funding, organization and boundaries, it is unlikely that any government is going to pursue the first option whatever the service advantages. Therefore, the second option, which looks at the process of decision-making for service delivery and planning, appears to be the more promising. This process approach will be explored more fully to find a way of working which shapes services in light of the experience of service-users and professionals alike.

The alternative approach proposed here is intended to apply to all agencies and interested parties involved in health and social care policy and practice. The purpose of the approach is twofold: to demonstrate that it is possible to establish mental health services which are not fragmented but planned and, second, to show that a systematic approach to individual care can be used to create an organizational audit to clarify service needs and service quality. This alternative process is comprised of seven steps which are set out below:

## SEVEN STEPS TO CHANGING SERVICES

### Step 1. Shared vision of services

Any process approach to care is dependent on there being a degree of agreement between the parties involved on the vision of the service to be provided. The key stake-holders in the mental health field are the purchasers of service, provider organizations, advocacy agencies, carers and service-users. To many people talk of 'vision' or 'mission statements' smacks of either wholly abstract ideas or a picture of idealistic motherhood and apple pie. But a vision of a service can be rooted in the daily experience of services and it can serve as a practical framework to concentrate on core tasks as well as principles of good practice. In Chapter 8 examples were given of one particular 'aims of service' paper used in inner-city Manchester which was practical and to which all involved could subscribe. However, one key requirement applies to vision statements if they are to prove to be robust: the agreement of the political leadership of the respective agencies. This ensures that at a later date when decisions on resources are taken they are informed by a common understanding of the aims of the service, the use of common outcome measures and the resources required to meet identified need. This point was well made by the commentators on the RWJ projects referred to in Chapter 7.

## Stage 2. Information system

If any approach to better coordinated user care is to be successful it is essential that there is reliable access to accurate information on the persons' circumstances, rather than some anecdotal information which may be based on opinion. However, the use of personal information on mental health service-users provokes a great deal of fear and anxiety, especially if that information is to be stored on computers. There is something of a double standard applied to users and professionals alike when comparing manual and automated information storage. The manual system may be more open to abuse and less reliable than new systems but it is often perceived as less threatening. The simple answer to this problem is to treat the patient database in the same way that a computerized personnel system would operate. This would mean that the service-user would have regular access to all the information held, which could be changed if factual errors occur. At the point at which a new user is referred to the service there are good practice and contractual reasons to record the persons' referral. Without this there is a significant risk that services will not be planned and delivered in a coordinated and thoughtful way. Without such a system there is a real danger that if the user has occasional involvement with services they will become discreet, isolated and fragmented episodes of care, rather than part of an overall service to the individual.

### Stage 3. Joint assessment

It is important that services are made available in a way which is appropriate to the individual; so for example a standardized assessment for residential accommodation is unlikely to be appropriate for a person who can live satisfactorily in the community. Equally, there is a pressing need to engage with the patient or client in seeking their agreement and participation in a planning process which claims to be for the individual. There is little point in seeking to complete a detailed assessment which would form the basis of a community care plan if the individual clearly expresses his/her opposition to the process. The purpose of the joint assessment is to bring together all of the stake-holders to consider a comprehensive range of information and opinion in order to form a plan to provide services.

### Stage 4. Joint agency meetings

The way in which the agencies meet to discuss the care of an individual of common interest is central to the whole process and there is a pressing need to agree joint formats and procedures for these discussions. There is already a precedent for this through the work on discharge arrangements established by the Mental Health Act under section 117 which requires clear plans to be made by the local authority in conjunction with health, for those patients who are about to leave hospital. One of the new features of joint assessment procedures is the appearance of the social services 'assessors' and 'case managers' who will effectively control access to social services support and coordinate services on the users' behalf. One of the possible implications of this arrangement is that social services may be represented at the joint agency meetings by the assessor who acts as a provider and the case manager as a purchaser.

## Stage 5. Service offered or unavailable

Having drafted an individual care plan through the joint agency meeting; established a lead person to overview the implementation of the plan, and coordinated the agencies' efforts, it is possible to produce a service plan which states what is needed by the user and what can be provided by whom. In a comprehensive service the range of services offered could include specialist psychiatric services; housing, leisure, income maintenance, advocates, domestic support and the relief for carers. Equally as important as offering services to meet the individual care plan is the recording of the shortfall between the ideal service and the service actually provided. This provides a practical way of building a picture of the needs of particular communities by aggregating the needs of individuals who present to specialist services. This is an alternative to the traditional epidemiological approach which is a poor proxy for mental health problems. There is a need for a parallel system which establishes the staff skills required to provide such services and an approach to staff development which arises from the experience of providing services for individual users. It is only when there is sufficient investment of time, energy and resources in staff development can there be a realistic expectation that quality mental health care will be part of the routine of service provision.

## Stage 6. Quality of life measures

One of the features of the fragmented services which are currently provided to service-users is the way in which agencies concentrate on measure of output from their agencies. It is common to provide returns to the Department of Health for the numbers of visits completed or the occupancy levels of particular types of accommodation. This data has little or nothing to do with the real-life problems of improving the quality of life of individual service-users. All services offered need to be part of a monitoring system which looks at the impact on the quality of life of the individual service-user through standardized questionnaires. With such an approach it is possible to build a joint agency picture of who does what and for whom. This information in turn can be reviewed and fed back into the overall information base which can be used to begin to build the community audit, matching the pattern of service provision with the known need.

## Stage 7. Review

The whole process of service provision from Stage 3 (joint assessment) to Stage 6 (quality of life measures) has to be capable of review and change. It is proposed that each service-user has a regular review which is fed back to both the joint agency meeting by the key worker and through the joint information base. In addition, the demographic, aggregated information on all service outcomes should be made available from the information system to the purchasers of services as part of the contract negotiation and monitoring process.

The seven-stage process set out above attempts to deal with some of the long-standing and new problems facing those who manage mental health care services. These issues include creating a shared vision of the service with stake-holders; common information systems, decisions on the appropriateness of services, service-user involvement, joint agency policies, individual care plans, monitoring of services required, quality of life measures, outcomes and staff development. The same process is set out in Figure 9.1.

This process is an alternative to long-established custom and practice on individual and service management and planning. For health, social services and service-users the old practices have served professionals and service alike – poorly. The approach outlined above is an attempt to overcome three particular problems which have dogged mental health services since the inception of the NHS:

1. Services have been developed in an information vacuum which has meant that concepts such as need have remained as abstract and unusable ideals. This approach seeks to record not only output of services but also outcomes on the quality of life for individuals.
2. Fragmented services have arisen from organizations which have coexisted, but failed to coordinate their activities; the development of a common vision agreed with purchasers of service would serve to bind together those working on the service-users' behalf.

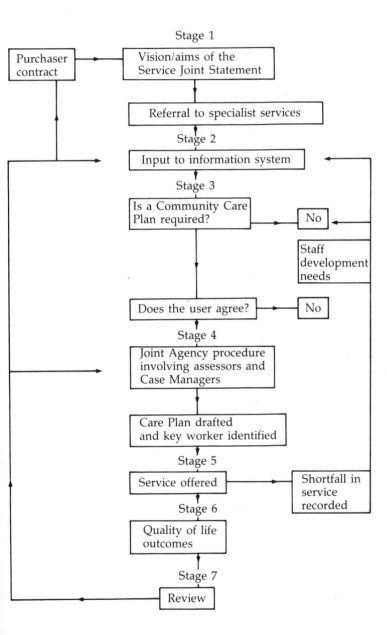

**Figure 9.1** Process model for specialist mental health services.

3.  The most important resource available to both health and social services is the people who work with and for the users. To date, the staff development needs of these people has been addressed separately from the provision of services. This approach looks to identify skills training and staff development as part of process of providing services itself, not as an isolated adjunct to it.

It is only when we can be explicit about the aims of our services and the particular model of services we seek to provide that we can begin to focus on the way in which we develop measures of outcome for the user. If the purpose of the service is to work to provide a range of services within a specialist mental health service then we need to recognize that this complex task cannot be done by a single agency in isolation from purchasers, other providers or the community within which it is based.

The approach to service development shown above is an attempt to turn on its head a traditional way of providing services, which assumes that the providers always know best and service provision is isolated from the consequences for the service-user. Undoubtedly it is easier and less challenging to make a set of decisions in isolation; to date this approach has produced services which are often seen as remote from both users' personal lives and their communities and separate from the political issues of policy and resources. This alternative approach rests on a number of simple assumptions: better information leads to better decisions; shared values are likely to produce more coherent services; need can be better assessed from the aggregated experience of those individuals who are referred to specialist services. Such an approach stands or falls on the capacity of those involved, from politicians to the service-users, to suspend willingly their disbelief that professionals are capable of working together in partnership with others in the community.

# 10

## Conclusion

This book has looked at the way in which society has responded to the mentally ill through public policy. In particular,
it has emphasized the shifts and changes in mental health
policy and practice and the way in which they relate to wider
changes in the society. Emphasis has been given to the
pathway between the past and the present in mental health
policy and the legacy of custom, practice and policy which has
been handed on over the last 200 years. It is often uncomfortable to recognize some of these links but 200 years after the
founding of 'The Retreat' it is likely that William Tuke would
recognize many of the weaknesses of provision for the mentally
ill in the 1990s.

### PUBLIC INSTITUTIONS AND THEIR PROBLEMS

Over the last 200 years there have been a number of strategies
developed to provide for the mentally ill which have dominated
the thinking of policy-makers and professionals alike. Chapters
1 and 2 traced the emergence of the public asylum out of the
eighteenth century arrangements which were informal, local
and haphazard. The asylums were created in a spirit of public
concern for the treatment of the mentally ill which resulted
from the reports of misuse and cruel treatment in the
workhouse, prison, old hospitals and the private madhouses.
The promise of the reformers who campaigned for the creation
of new public asylums was to provide humane, well-regulated,
economic and effective provision for the mentally ill. The
asylums were not intended to treat mental illness, but to
contain the mentally ill. The wider significance of the reform

of provision for 'lunatics' was to be found in the way in which it illustrated the potential for the development of publicly-managed institutions. These new institutions were seen by those involved in the reform movement as powerful expressions of the idea of 'good government'. What resulted was the creation of institutions which took little account of the individual needs of the asylum population. Over time the ideal of care was replaced with the routine of the institution itself. Ironically it is debatable if the majority of the asylum residents were actually mentally ill, as the new institutions were principally used to house one part of the pauper population.

Within three decades of their creation the asylums became places of fear and loathing; with this people with mental illness were set aside from society at large as a group of troubled and troublesome people best kept behind the walls of the asylum. The old fears of being mistreated in the private madhouses was replaced with a moral panic about being wrongfully detained in the asylum. This created a demand for a new policy by the end of the nineteenth century which required people being admitted to the asylums to be certified as lunatics before they could be admitted. This policy in turn became one of the major obstacles to the development of mental health policy up to the creation of the NHS in 1948.

People with mental illness were caught in a terrible paradox as all provision was based in the asylums; no sane person would conceivably wish to be admitted and therefore to be certified and admitted resulted in the individual being branded as mad. The asylums were built and filled with a range of people, most of whom were pauper lunatics. In time, the institutions became one of a variety of forms of disposals for the magistrates and other public officials. This resulted in a dual legacy for the mentally ill and for those who worked in the asylums. The first part of this legacy consisted of the range of large asylums themselves which housed people with mental illness and which have continued in use. The second part of the legacy was the set of attitudes which were associated with life in the asylums and which in turn led to the sense of stigma carried by the mentally ill. In many respects this proved to be both the most enduring and most corrosive of the two legacies, as it informed public and private opinion alike.

Much of the work of those who argued for mental health reforms has been an attempt to undo this Victorian legacy which proved so persistent. The asylums and the use of certification was a response to a set of contemporary problems which brought about new powers for government and further estranged those people who failed to cope with daily life. It is important that we see the nineteenth century reforms in their own context. The building of the asylums and the creations of the lunacy laws were honest attempts to improve the provision for people with mental illness. These policies, however, were to result in enormous personal cost for those who were subject to institutional life. It is easy for us to look critically at these developments and feel that the policies and practices were based on ignorance and fear. However a case can be made that the efforts to move away from the asylums has been informed by at least as much over-confidence and dogma expressed by those who sought to close the asylums as by those who originally campaigned for their construction.

## THE SEARCH FOR ALTERNATIVES

Chapters 3 and 4 critically reviewed the alternatives to the old hospitals and highlighted the confusion which surrounded community care. The concept of community care seemed to have almost universal appeal as it appeared to promise both the closure of the old asylums and the provision of cheaper alternatives in the community. Unfortunately, it was the very breadth of the concept which proved to be its central weakness. There is no common agreement between policy-makers or politicians of the left or the right as to what is meant by community care or the implications of such a policy. The concept is a fine and well-used rhetorical tool for any argument, whether it is to condemn all hospital care as repressive; to argue that it means abandoning the mentally ill in the community without support or it is the vehicle for a more independent life free from the problems of institutions.

Over the last 30 years there have been a number of strategies and solutions developed to take the place of the asylums. These alternatives range from the medical 'revolution' of the 1950s to the unfulfilled promises of well-resourced community mental health services. Chapters 4 and 5 looked at the health and social care policy alternatives which appeared in the unlikely shape of a radical conservative government at the end of the 1970s with the first Thatcher administration. The significance of the Thatcher years was that they sought to look again at the fundamental questions raised in the nineteenth century concerning the 'proper' relationship between government and the individual. The key question was how much should the government intervene in the lives of its citizens and provide a range of publicly-funded services. This produced a range of policies, many of which were drawn from the American health care market, informed by a belief in deregulation and a commitment to the market place as a way of regulating human behaviour and choices. What resulted was a wholesale re-think about the place of public services and the provision of health services. In turn, the organization of health and social care was radically altered and driven by the separation of purchaser and provider functions. The experience of the market place was brought in to regulate these relationships through the use of contracts for services.

The early 1980s saw an economic recession replaced by a business boom and the growth of the service sector taking the place of traditional manufacturing in Britain. Many people prospered but people with mental health problems became marginal to mainstream society. A society increasingly driven by the market place and the desire to generate personal wealth held few choices for people with mental illness, who too often found the challenge of finding a place to live an overwhelming burden. The old hospitals continued to be run down, both in terms of the total numbers of patients overall as well as the living conditions for those long-stay patients who remained. The community care initiatives promised the appropriate services to all: irrespective of their circumstances, or the resources or skills available to meet them. To those who needed hospital care it promised the development of smaller and better accommodation and services which could be funded through land sales of the old hospital sites. To those people who moved in to the community it promised personal freedom, but all too often the community was either hostile or indifferent. The preservation of the old hospitals for those patients who were not resettled and the development of new community services for those who were, had to be funded simultaneously from the same pot of money. Resources were to be transferred with the patients involved in community resettlement through the allocation of 'dowries'. The purchasing power of this money dwindled rapidly during the late 1980s and early 1990s as inflation took effect and skilled labour costs rose.

The reforms of the early 1990s contained within them a number of notable features which potentially promised better services for the mentally ill. In particular the development of a care programme approach; case management, service-user participation, outcome measures and a renewed emphasis on domiciliary services. The unspoken part of the policy was the failure to fund these developments and the contraction in social services and income maintenance funding. It is perhaps too early to tell if more than the promise will be sustained, but the initial signs suggest that caution is required. The real winner has been the rhetoric of the politicians of all parties who fuelled expectations, yet fail to deliver.

## THE PROMISE OF INTEGRATED SERVICES

The debates between hospital versus community provision has proved itself ultimately to be sterile and diverting. There is much evidence to suggest that a range of services are required from highly intensive ward-based services to user-defined community support programmes. Resources are locked up in a number of ways, in old hospitals which have little value to new patients and in a variety of un-coordinated agencies.

Chapter 7 examined some of the American mental health experience, in particular those innovative demonstration projects which have attempted to deal with the problem of fragmented services. However, there is a central irony to the American health story. Much of the market-drive ideas which informed the Thatcher reforms in Britain were derived from the management of American health care industry, at a time when that country was actively looking for a proper *system* of health care itself. As Britain looked to America as a business-like model for health purchasing and delivery, so America looked to Britain as an example of quality services with controlled costs. If there is any one lesson from the American experience it is that change can only succeed when professionals achieve a common vision which can be shared by the politicians and policy-makers within the key agencies.

Chapter 8 turned to the experience of one inner city district in Britain in order to look at the local impact of the wider changes in health and social care. This case study of central Manchester sought to bring together the clinical and mangerial issues which informed the discussions on the health reforms of the 1990s. Whilst it is important to create an organization which has a clear structure for decision-making it is of equal importance to work on the process issues. Services are not created solely through an administrative reform as they result from the application of a variety of skills brought to bear on a common problem. In the same sense the changes in health and social care provide an opportunity for local innovation and experiment.

## UNFULFILLED PROMISES

At the heart of the changes in health and social care is the organizational separation of the purchaser and the provider. This change gives the responsibility for the assessment health needs to the District Health Authorities and social needs to the local authority Social Services Department. However, the assessment of individual need is the responsibility of the particular professional in each agency, whereas responsibility for the global needs of the population rest with the agency. This tension will be difficult to resolve in a number of ways: for example, needs may be identified but not met because of a failure to agree a common value base on which to judge priorities. If the experience of health and social services over the last two decades is a guide, then people with mental illness will continue to be the poor relation to other care groups. There is no evidence on which to draw any other conclusion, as to date both health and social services have failed to meet their responsibilities for the mentally ill in three key areas:

1. Health services and local authorities have failed to establish a joint vision of the service they wish to see.
2. Without a shared set of aims it is not difficult to fail to fund adequate services.

3. Quite simply both major public agencies have demonstrably failed to prove that they can work together for the mutual benefit of the service-user.

Yet out of this picture of fragmented services, poorly resourced provision, beset with political inertia there is the possibility for change for the better. In Chapter 9 an alternative approach for the development of a new way of working was explored in order to inform the process of care decision-making and giving. The relationship between cost and quality of service is increasingly taking centre stage in the policy debates on health and social care through the use of service contracts between purchasers and providers. Much of the discussion continues to focus on the internal detail of service standards or industrial type quality standards rather than the impact services have on the quality of life of individual service-users. Equally, there is little real understanding of the economic, social or personal cost of mental illness, because all too often it is regarded as an acceptable or unmeasured cost which may only be borne by the individual service-user or their immediate carers. It is even difficult to calculate the costs of providing the range of necessary mental health services for a locality as the information is spread amongst a variety of sources. These issues have to be tackled before any sustainable account of the relationship between cost, quality and outcomes can be made. In the meantime, services are all too often a function of the quality of personal relationships between professionals in differing agencies. Such an approach provides no way of accounting for either cost or quality measures.

## GOOD PRACTICE AND BAD PLANNING

There are many examples of excellent local initiatives established between service-users, health authorities, social services, the voluntary sector and carers. But this must not be confused with the wider problems of the parent organizations' failure to work together. Many of the excellent collaborations which have developed are as a result of a shared understanding of the common problem of trying to make the system work for the individual service-user; not because of the exaltations of central government or the obstacles presented by the key agencies.

Out of the direct experience of managing and providing care for individuals it is possible to construct an alternative model of a mental health system which works for the service-user and professional alike, as a by product of inter-agency collaboration. Such an approach was set out in Chapter 9 as an alternative to the traditional ways of assessing needs and managing services. The two key features of this approach are the common experience of professionals and service-users and the 'bottom-up' approach to decision-making. One of the benefits of the approach is that it does not polarize individual assessment of needs and the overall needs of the areas population. The use of an agreed process for decision-making, the central roles of information and continued professional development mark this approach as an alternative. Without radical alternatives the risk is that services will continue to be unplanned and delivered in an atmosphere of organizational feuding. It is this feuding and the fragmented services it generates which has characterized much of the discussion on the implementation of the community care reforms.

If mental health services are to change for the better then the measure of that change must be the degree to which they can help improve the quality of life of individual service-users. There is a sad circularity in the history of services for the mentally ill, which results time and time again in the service-user being the focus of heated debates on social policy and professional practice. Every few years new panaceas are presented to the 'problem' of the mentally ill. All too often these 'solutions' are in response to crisis in provision. These solutions fail to give those who provide services either the resources or the support they require and those who need services the facilities they require.

Central government announced the intention in *The Health of the Nation* (1991) to close the remaining 90 large psychiatric hospitals before the year 2000. The Department of Health has made it a target in the consultative paper that it will look to develop district services further. But what does this really mean? The key resources required are skilled staff, suitable venues in which to deliver services and the cooperation of a number of other agencies who manage non-health services.

For the user of mental health services, both in hospital and the community, help appears all to often to be fragmented, confusing and occasionally hostile. This fragmentation results from the unevenness of services which have been chronically under-funded and organized through separate agencies who share no common processes of culture. One result is that people with mental health problems are shuffled from agency to agency and all too often are re-classified according to the needs of the particular organization. Consequently, people with mental health problems become part of the homeless or become lost in the petty offending populations of the prison system. There is a new revolving door in mental health services especially for the long-term mentally ill who move between homelessness, prisons, hospitals and residential care in a way that is reminiscent of the nineteenth century provision. Residential care could so easily become the new private madhouses of the twentieth century, especially when the responsibility for funding is transferred from social security to the local authority. The prospects for regular inspections, monitoring and the integration of services are likely to be all the more remote given the reduced funding of many local authority social services departments.

## IMPROVING INDIVIDUALS' QUALITY OF LIFE

The need for an alternative strategy is not a preferred option for mental illness services, it is an essential prerequisite for the provision of an acceptable basic service which seeks to improve the quality of life of individuals who live with mental illness. Service-users, be they patients of the NHS or clients of the social services care little about which agency does what; their principal concern is that somebody will respond appropriately to his or her needs at that time. Brandon (1991) in his work on consumer power in psychiatric services questions the basis of current mental health provision and asks for whom it works? What is clear from Brandon's book is that the idea of consumer power means far more than greater user involvement; it is essentially about the power relationships between public agencies such as the health and social services and those they provide for.

Despite Britain's two centuries of experience in developing public policy for people with mental illness, for many mental health service-users powerlessness has become a way of life. A better quality of life continues to remain an aspiration rather than a reality.

# References

Audit Commission (1986) *Making a Reality of Community Care*, HMSO, London.

Barton, R. (1959) *Institutional Neurosis*, John Wright, Bristol.

Beecham, J., Knapp, M. and Fenyo, A. (1991) *Costs, Needs and Outcomes: Community Care for People with Long-Term Mental Health Problems*, Discussion Paper 730/2 PSSRU, University of Kent.

Bigelow, D.A., Bodsky, G., Steward, L. and Osborn, M. (1982) 'The Concept and Measurement of Quality of Life', in Stahler, G.J. and Task, W.R. (eds) *Innovative Approaches to Mental Health*, pp. 345–366. Academic Press, New York.

Brandon, D. (1991) *Consumer Power in Psychiatric Services*, Macmillan Education, London.

British Medical Association (1987) *Deprivation and Ill Health*, London Board of Science and Education.

Butler, T. (1985) *Mental Health, Social Policy and the Law*, Macmillan, London.

Butler, T. (1990) 'Care out of Control' *The Health Service Journal*, 23rd August, 1250–1.

Butler, T. (1991) 'Working Together – results and prospects' *Caring for People*, Department of Health, London, No. 3, 4–5.

Butler, T. and Thomas, P . (1990) 'Changing Practices in Mental Health Care: A lesson from America' *Psychiatric Bulletin*, **14**, 730–732.

Central Manchester Health Authority (1989) *People Poverty and Health*, unpublished paper.

Central Manchester Health Authority (1990) *The Health of Central Manchester*, unpublished paper.

Central Manchester Joint Planning Team for Mental Health (1990) *Report to the Joint Care Planning Team,*, unpublished paper.

Clifford, P. and Craig, T. (1989) *Case Management systems for the Long-Term Mentally Ill*, National Unit for Psychiatric Research and Development, London.

Creed, F., Black, D., Anthony, P. *et al*. 'Randomised Control Trial of Day and In-Patient Psychiatric Treatment 2: Comparison of Two

Hospitals' *British Journal of Psychiatry* **158**, 183–189.

Dean, C. and Gadd, E.M. (1990) 'Home Treatment for Acute Mental Illness' *British Medical Journal* **31**, 1021–1027.

Department of Health (1975) *Better Services for the Mentally Ill*, HMSO, London.

Department of Health (1986) *Mental Health Statistics for England*, HMSO, London.

Department of Health (1987) *Promoting Better Health*, HMSO, London.

Department of Health (1989a) *Caring for People*, HMSO, London.

Department of Health (1989b) *Working for Patients*, HMSO, London.

Department of Health (1989c) Personal Social Services: Provision for Mentally Ill in England 1977–1987, *Statistical Bulletin*, **3**, 89.

Department of Health (1990) The Care Programme Approach for people with a mental illness referred to specialist psychiatric services, *HC(90)23*, HMSO, London.

Department of Health (1991a) *The Health of the Nation, a Consultation Document for Health in England*, HMSO, London.

Department of Health (1991b) *Services for people with a severe mental illness: review in progress and problems in implementing the 1975 White Paper 'Better Services for the Mentally Ill'*, HMSO, London.

Department of Health (1991c) *The Patients' Charter*, HMSO, London.

Department of Health and Social Services Inspectorate (1991) *Care Management and Assessment: Practitioners' Guide Care Management and Assessment: Managers' Guide Care Management and Assessment: Summary of Practice Guidance* HMSO, London.

Department of Health and Welsh Office (1990)*Code of Practice: Mental Health Act 1989*, HMSO, London.

Department of Social Security (1989) *Social Security Statistics*, HMSO, London.

Engels, F. (1892) *The Condition of the working class in England in 1844*, George Allen and Unwin, London.

Foucault, M. (1967) *Madness and Civilization – A History of Insanity in the Age of Reason*, Tavistock, London.

Goffman, E. (1961) *Asylums: Essays in the social situation of mental patients and other inmates*, Phean, Harmondsworth, UK.

Goldman, H., Adams, N.H. and Taube, C.A. (1983) 'De-institutionalisation: demythologised' *Hospital and Community Psychiatry*, **34**, 129–134.

Goldman, H.H. and Morrisey, J.P. and Klerman, (1985) 'The Alchemy of Mental Health Policy: Homelessness and the south cycle of reform' *American Journal of Public Health*, **75**, 727–731.

Goldman, H.H., Lehman , A., Morrisey, J.P. *et al.* (1990a) 'Design for the National evaluation of the Robert Wood Johnson Foundaton programme on chronic mental illness' *Hospital and Community Psychiatry*, **41** (11), 1217.

Goldman, H.H., Morrisey, J.P. and Ridgely, M.S. (1990b) *The Robert Wood Johnson Foundation Programme on Chronic Mental Illness: Interview findings from the site level evaluation*, unpublished paper.

Goldberg, D. and Huxley, P. (1980) *Mental Illness in the Community:*

*The pathway to Psychiatric Care,* Tavistock Publication, London.

Griffiths, R. (1983) *NHS Management Enquiry Report,* DHSS, London.

Health Care Cost Containment Council (1989) *The First Hospital Effectiveness Report,* Harrisburg, Pennsylvania, USA.

Hudson, B. (1989) 'Collaboration: the elusive chimera' *The Health Service Journal,* 19th January, 82–83.

Huxley, P. (1990) 'Effective case management for mentally ill people: the relevence of recent evidence from the U.S.A. for case management in the United Kingdom.' *Social Work and Social Science Review,* **2**(3), 192–203.

Joint Committee on Mental Illness and Health (1961) *Action for Mental Health,* Science Edition, New York.

Jones, K. (1972) *A history of mental health services,* Routledge and Kegan Paul, London.

Jones, K. (1988) *Experience in Metal Health – Community Care and Social Policy,* Sage, London.

Jowell, T. (1991) *Policy in practice – Conference paper* Department of Health, London.

Kiesler, C.A. (1982) 'Public and Professional Myths about Mental Hospitalisation: an Empirical Re-assessment of Policy Related Beliefs'. *American Psychology,* **37,** 1323–1339.

Kingsley, S. and Towell, D. (1989) *Designing local processes for service development,* King's Fund working paper, London.

Knapp, M. and Beecham, J. (1990) 'Costing Mental Health Services' *Psychological Medicine* **20,** 893–908.

Knapp, M., Beecham, J., Anderson, J. *et al.* (1990) 'The Taps Projects: Predicting the community care costs of closing mental hospitals' *British Journal of Psychiatry,* **157,** 661–670.

Lehman , A.F. (1983) 'The well-being of chronic mental patients *Archives of General Psychiatry,* **40,** 369–377.

Lehman, A.F. (1988) 'A quality of life interview of the chronically mentally ill' *Evaluations and Programme Planning,* **11,** 51–62.

Lehman, A.F., Possidente, S. and Hawker, F. (1986) 'The quality of life of chronic patients in a state hospital and in Community residences' *Hospital and Community Psychiatry* **37,** 9.

Manchester City Council (1986) *Health Inequalities and Manchester,* unpublished paper.

Manchester City Council (1988) *Poverty in Manchester – the third investigation,* unpublished paper.

Manchester City Council (1989) *Poverty in Manchester: The third investigation,* unpublished paper.

Manchester Joint Consultative Committee (1986)    Health Inequalities in Manchester, unpublished paper.

Mental Health Foundation (1990) *Mental Illness: The fundamental facts* MHF, London.

Ministry of Health (1962) *A Hospital plan for England and Wales,* Cmnd 1604, HMSO, London.

Mosher, L.R. (1983) 'Alternatives to Psychiatric Hospitalization: Why has Research Failed to be Translated into Practice'. *The New*

*England Journal of Medicine,* **309**(25), 1579–1580.

Office of Population, Census and Statistics (1986) *Population Statistics and General Household Survey,* HMSO, London.

Offices of Population, Census and Statistics (1990) *Population Statistics and General Household Survey,* HMSO, London.

Oliver, J. (1991) 'The social care directive: development of a quality of life profile for use in community services for the mentally ill' *Social Work and Social Science Review,* **3**(1).

Roland *et al.* (1989) 'Community Care: Agenda for Action a response from the National Demonstration services in psychiatric Rehabilitation' *Psychiatric Bulletin* , **13**, 538–541.

Rosenberger, J.W. (1990) 'Central Mental Health Services: politically flawed?' *Hospital and Community Psychiatry,* **41**(11), 1171.

Rothman, D.J. (1971) The Discovery of the Asylum: social order and disorder in the New Republic. Little, Brown and Co., Boston, MA.

Ryan, P. Ford, R. and Clifford, P. (1991) *Case Management and Community Care,* Research and Development for Psychiatry, London.

Scull, A.T. (1975) 'From Madness to Mental Illness' *Archives Europeannes de Sociologie,* **16**.

Scull, A.T. (1979) *'Museums of Madness: The Social Organisation of Insanity in Nineteenth-Century England,* Allen Lane, London.

Shepherd, G. (1990) Case Management. *Health Trends* Vol 22, No. 2.

Shore, M.F. and Cohen, M. (1990) 'The Robert Wood Johnson Foundation Programme on chronic mental illness: An Overview' *Hospital and Community Psychiatry,* **41**(11), 1212.

Social Services Inspectorate (1990) *All Change: From hospital to Community,* Department of Health, London.

Stein, L.I. and Test, M.A. (1980) 'Alternatives to mental hospital treatment: Conceptual model, treatment programme and clinical evaluation' *Archives of General Psychiatry,* **37**, 292–397.

Talbott, J.A. (1978) *The Death of the Asylum: A Critical Study of State Hospital Management, Services and Care.* Grune and Stratton, New York.

Tooth and Brooke (1961) 'Trends in the Mental Hospital population and their effect on future planning' *Lancet* , **i**, 1710.

Towell, D. and Thomas, D. (1989) *Lessons from America,* unpublished paper.

Warner, R. (1985) *Recovery from Schizophrenia: Psychiatry and Political Economy.* Routledge and Kegan Paul, London.

Willenbring, M.L., Ridgely, M.S., Stinchfield, S. and Rose, M. (1990) *Application of Case Management in Alcohol and Drug Dependency: Matching techniques and Populations,* Publication no. ADM 91–1766, National Institute on Alcohol Abuse and Alcoholism, Rockville, MD, USA.

Wing, J.K. (1990) 'The function of Asylum' *British Journal of Psychiatry* **157**, 822–827.

# Index